The Endocrinology of Aging

The Endocrinology of Aging

Editors

W. A. Scherbaum · W. G. Rossmanith

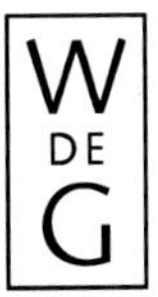

Walter de Gruyter
Berlin · New York 1995

Editors

Prof. Dr. W. A. Scherbaum
Universitätsklinikum Leipzig
Medizinische Klinik und Poliklinik III
Ph.-Rosenthal-Str. 27
D-04103 Leipzig
Germany

PD Dr. W. G. Rossmanith
Universitäts-Frauenklinik
Prittwitzstr. 40
D-89075 Ulm
Germany

Die Deutsche Bibliothek − Cataloging-in-Publication Data

The **endocrinology of aging** / Ed. W. A. Scherbaum ; W. G. Rossmanith. −
Berlin ; New York : de Gruyter, 1995
   ISBN 3-11-014591-X
   NE: Scherbaum, Werner [Hrsg.]

List of first-mentioned contributors

PD L. Duntas, M. D.
Leoforos Pendelis 95
Halandri 15234
Athens
Greece

Prof. H. L. Fehm, M. D.
Klinik für Innere Medizin
Universität zu Lübeck
Ratzeburger Allee 160
D-23562 Lübeck
Germany

Prof. J. Hensen, M. D.
Medizinische Klinik I
Universität Erlangen – Nürnberg
Krankenhausstr. 12
D-91054 Erlangen
Germany

PD Dipl. Psych. I. Heuser, M. D.
Max-Planck-Institut für Psychiatrie
Deutsche Forschungsanstalt für Psychiatrie
Klinisches Institut
Kraepelinstr. 10
D-80804 München
Germany

Prof. W. Kerner, M. D.
Klinik für Innere Medizin
Universität zu Lübeck
Ratzeburger Allee 160
D-23562 Lübeck
Germany

Prof. (em.) Ch. Lauritzen, M. D.
Alpenstr. 49
D-89075 Ulm
Germany

Prof. (em.) J. Meites, Ph. D.
Michigan State University
Giltner Hall
East Lansing, Michigan, 48824-1101
USA

PD W. G. Rossmanith, M. D.
Universitäts-Frauenklinik
Prittwitzstr. 40
D-89075 Ulm
Germany

Prof. W. A. Scherbaum, M. D.
Universitätsklinikum Leipzig
Zentrum für Innere Medizin
Medizinische Klinik III
Ph.-Rosenthal-Str. 27
D-04103 Leipzig
Germany

Prof. D. F. Swaab, M. D.
The Netherlands Institute for Brain Research
Meibergdreef 33
1105 AZ Amsterdam ZO
The Netherlands

Prof. J. D. Veldhuis, M. D.
Division of Endocrinology and Metabolism
Health Sciences Center
University of Virginia
Charlottesville, Virginia 22908
USA

Prof. A. Vermeulen, M. D.
Department of Endocrinology
University Hospital of Ghent
De Pintelaan 186
9000 Ghent
Belgium

Ch.-F. Wolf, M. D.
Institut für Klinische Chemie
Universität Ulm
Robert-Koch-Str. 8
D-89070 Ulm
Germany

PD Chr. Wüster, M. D.
Abteilung Innere Medizin I
Medizinische Klinik der Universität Heidelberg
Bergheimer Straße 58
D-69115 Heidelberg
Germany

Prof. R. Ziegler, M. D.
Abteilung Innere Medizin I
Medizinische Klinik der Universität Heidelberg
Bergheimer Straße 58
D-69115 Heidelberg
Germany

Preface

The endocrinology of aging deserves special attention from several points of view. While some biological functions, such as fasting blood glucose, remain unchanged during the lifespan of normal individuals, other parameters such as glucose tolerance tend to deteriorate in old age. The most dramatic physiological endocrine changes affect the gonadal function of women when the menopause marks the end of reproductive years. Also, male fertility continuously decreases over the years.

The percentage of elderly people is rapidly increasing in the Western world and also in other regions. As a consequence, we will face more age-associated diseases in the forthcoming years. While in 1990 about four million people in the U.S.A. were over age 85, this number will increase to eight million in 2010 and to over twenty million in the year 2050. According to an epidemiological calculation, the prevalence of non-insulin dependent diabetes mellitus — which is rapidly increasing in advanced age — will rise between 1990 and 2000 in India from 15 to 35 million people, in the People's Republic of China from 6 to 15 million, in Africa from 7 to 20 million and in the U.S.A. from 8 to 15 million people. This will have a major socio-economic impact, with consequences for health care strategies.

Diagnostic procedures and therapeutic approaches to disease states may be different in the elderly as compared to young individuals. To define the goals for therapeutic intervention, illness should be clearly distinguished from age-associated changes. To accomplish this, signs and symptoms of diseases have to be assessed and defined, particularly in the elderly. A well-known example is monosymptomatic or oligosymptomatic hyperthyroidism which mainly occurs in old age and represents a diagnostic challenge. As a consequence, the clinician will depend on biochemical tests to confirm or exclude the diagnosis. However, correct interpretation of hormone values in the elderly requires special attention.

At present about 40% of drugs in the Western world are consumed by patients over the age of 65 years. Due to multimorbidity, the number of drugs and thus, the risk of drug interaction, increase in old age. Metabolism and renal elimination of many drugs are reduced in the elderly. It is therefore not surprising that side effects of drugs are three times more frequent in elderly compared with young individuals. This notion is relevant to the therapeutic strategy in old age. It should focus on the most relevant individual disabilities, always bearing in mind the biological age and the life expectancy of an aged individual.

This volume intends to offer a selection of both research-orientated endocrinology and practical aspects as to the diagnosis and treatment of endocrine diseases in the elderly. We wish to express our gratitude and appreciation to all the authors who contributed to this book offering a profound insight into their special fields of research and clinical practice.

Leipzig and Ulm, January 1995

Werner A. Scherbaum   Winfried G. Rossmanith

Contents

x   Contents

The human hypothalamus in aging and dementia

D. F. Swaab

Recent research into the human hypothalamus has revealed a number of morphological and functional changes during the process of aging and in Alzheimer's disease, the most common cause of dementia. There is a causal relationship, at least partly, between these alterations and the well-known changes in functions observed during, e. g. sleep disturbances, restlessness, diminished sexual activity, changes in eating behavior and metabolism, activation of the adrenal system, mood changes and menopausal flushes. Quite a few of the alterations observed in the hypothalamic nuclei during aging and in Alzheimer's disease are caused by changes outside this brain structure: the visual system in the case of the suprachiasmatic nucleus, kidney changes in the case of the supraoptic and paraventricular nucleus and changes in sex hormone levels in the case of the arcuate nucleus. This offers the exciting possibility of influencing the aging process of this part of the brain by correcting the neural and hormonal input of the hypothalamus.

1 Suprachiasmatic nucleus

The suprachiasmatic nucleus (SCN) is a small structure (0.25 mm^3) that is considered to be the major circadian pacemaker of the mammalian brain, coordinating hormonal and behavioral circadian rhythms [46]. In conventionally thionine-stained sections the human SCN cannot be recognized with certainty and therefore immunocytochemical labelling of the nucleus is necessary [61]. The shape of the human SCN is sexually dimorphic, i. e. more elongated in women and more spherical in men, but the vasopressin cell number and volume are similar in both sexes [58]. Neurons that are immunoreactive for vasopressin, vasoactive intestinal polypeptide (VIP), neuropeptide-Y and neurotensin are present in the SCN in a particular anatomical organization [36, 38]. Typical for the human SCN, as compared to monkeys and other animals, are (1) the very large population of neurotensin cells and (2) the large population of NPY neurons obscuring a geneticulo-hypothalamic tract − if such a tract is present in the human brain at all [38]. Recent observations have revealed a marked seasonal variation in the volume and cell number of the human SCN in relation to the variations in photoperiod; values were twice as high in autumn as in summer [22]. Similar circadian fluctuations were observed in the SCN of young adults (Hofman and Swaab, unpubl. results). A lesion in the suprachiasmatic region of the anterior hypothalamus, e. g. as the result of a tumor, indeed results in disturbed circadian rhythmus in humans [53, 7]. Totally blind people may show free-running temperature, cortisol and melatonin rhythms. In addition, they may suffer from sleep disturbances [47]. These observations underscore the importance of the light-dark cycle for synchronisation and of the SCN for circadian rhythms in humans.

Recent morphometric analysis of the SCN in 10 homosexual men revealed that the volume of this nucleus was 1.7 times as large as that of a reference group of 18 male subjects, and that it contained 2.1 times as many cells [62]. It might be that programmed postnatal cell death, usually occurring from 13−16 months after birth onwards, is limited in homosexual men. In 3 male to female transsexuals extreme values were observed in the SCN and SDN. It is not yet clear what the functional implications of this findings might be, although there are various indications that the SCN is involved in aspects of sexual behavior and reproduction [59].

Age-related changes in circadian rhythms have been reported in humans as well as in non-human species [71]. A fragmentation of sleep-wake patterns occurs in senescence, a phenomenon that is even more pronounced in Alzheimer's disease [37, 75, 42]. In Alzheimer's disease the disruptions of the circadian rhythms are often so severe that they lead to hospitalization of the elderly [49] and are even thought to contribute to mental decline [11]. For this reason the number of cells in the SCN was determined during aging and in Alzheimer's disease. A marked decrease was found in SCN total cell number and in the number of vasopressin-expressing neurons in subjects of 80−100 years of age, while in Alzheimer's disease these changes were even more dramatic [58, 58] Cytoskeletal alterations have also been found in the SCN of Alzheimer patients [64]. With respect to the degenerative changes of the SCN it may be important to note that both the retina and the optic nerve, which provide direct and indirect light input to the SCN, show degenerative changes in Alzheimer's disease [19, 65, 28]. In addition to degenerative changes, Alzheimer patients are generally exposed to less light than their age-matched controls [5]. As a result, both the input of the visual system to the SCN and the SCN itself seem to be seriously affected in Alzheimer's disease. The contribution of each of these components to circadian disturbances has yet to be investigated. Preliminary observations [40] show that behavioral disorders such as wandering, agitation or delirium almost disappeared, and that sleep-wake rhythm disorders improved in Alzheimer patients following exposure to bright light for two hours per morning. This indicates that stimulation of the SCN might have important therapeutic consequences.

2 Sexually dimorphic nucleus (intermediate nucleus, INAH-1)

The sexually dimorphic nucleus of the preoptic area (SDN) was first described in the rat brain by Gorski et al. [16]. Due to differences in perinatal steroid levels, the SDN in the male rat is 3−8 times larger than in the female rat [27]. On the basis of lesion experiments in rats, it was found that the SDN seems to be involved in aspects of male sexual behavior, i.e. mounting, intro-mission and ejaculation [66, 8]. However, the effects of lesions on sexual behavior are only slight, so it may well be that the major functions of the SDN are still unknown at present.

The SDN in the young adult human brain is twice as large in males (0.20 mm^3) as in females (0.10 mm^3) and contains twice as many cells [57]. The SDN is located between the supraoptic and paraventricular nucleus at the same rostro-caudal level as the suprachiasmatic nucleus. The SDN is identical to the "intermediate nucleus" described by Braak and Braak [3], and to the INAH-1 of Allen et al. [2]. In the human brain, sexual dimorphism is not present at birth. At that moment, cell numbers are similar in boys and girls and the SDN contains no more than 20% of the number of cells found around 2−4 years of age. From birth up to this age, cell numbers increase equally rapidly in both sexes. A sex difference does not occur until about the fourth year postnatally, when cell numbers start to decrease in girls, whereas in males they remain stable until approximately 50 years of age, when they rapidly decrease. In females a second phase of marked cell loss sets in after the age of 70 (Fig. 1) [60, 20]. The sharp decrease in cell numbers in the SDN later in life might be related to the dramatic hormonal changes which accompany both male and female senescence [20], and to the decrease in male sexual activity [72]. It is not clear whether the hormonal changes are cause or effect of the observed cell loss in this nucleus. Cell numbers in the SDN of Alzheimer's disease patients were found to be within the normal range for age and sex [60].

A prominent theory is that sexual orientation develops as a result of an interaction between the developing brain and sex hormones [10, 15]. According to Dörner's hypothesis, male homosexuals have a female differentiation of the hypothalamus. This theory was not supported by our data on the SDN in homosexual men. Neither the SDN volume nor the cell numbers of homosexual men who died of AIDS differed from that of the male reference groups in the same age range, nor from that of heterosexuals also suffering from AIDS [60, 62]. The fact that no difference in SDN cell number was observed between homo- and heterosexual men who had died of AIDS refutes the general formulation of Dörner's hypothesis that male homosexuals have "a female hypothalamus".

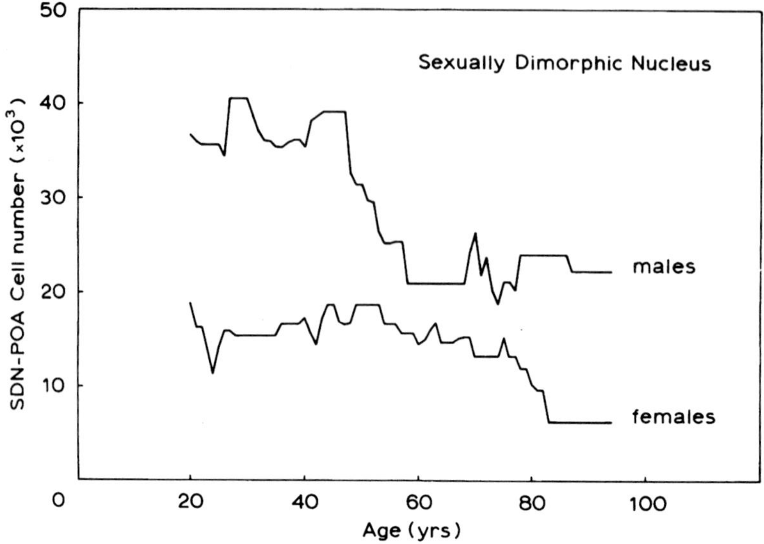

Fig. 1 Age-related changes in the total cell number of the sexually dimorphic nucleus of the preoptic area (SDN-POA) in the human hypothalamus. The general trend in the data is enhanced by using smoothed growth curves. Note that in males SDN-POA cell number steeply declines between the age of 50–60 years, whereas in females a more gradual cell loss is observed around the age of 80 years. These curves demonstrate that the reduction in cell number in the human SDN-POA in senescence is a non-linear, sex-dependent process. (From Hofman and Swaab, 1989, with permission.)

In Alzheimer's disease — not in controls — SDN neurons and dystrophic neurites are stained with cytoskeletal markers such as Alz-50, anti-tau, anti-paried helical filaments and anti-ubiquitin, in spite of the fact that there is no difference in SDN cell numbers between Alzheimer patients and controls [64].

3 Supraoptic and paraventricular nucleus and accessory nuclei

The large neurosecretory cells of the hypothalamic supraoptic and paraventricular nucleus (SON and PVN) produce the neuropeptides vasopressin and oxytocin which are released into the blood circulation in the neurohypophysis. Vasopressin acts as an anti-diuretic hormone on the kidney and in women oxytocin is involved in labor and lactation. Parvocellular vasopressin neurons of the PVN project into the brain and influence central processes [14]. Oxytocin has central effects for example food intake (see below), maternal and reproductive behavior [25] and in males might be involved in sexual arousal and ejaculation [39].

The neurons of the SON and PVN form a population of extremely stable cells in normal aging and in Alzheimer's disease; no loss in neurons or total cell

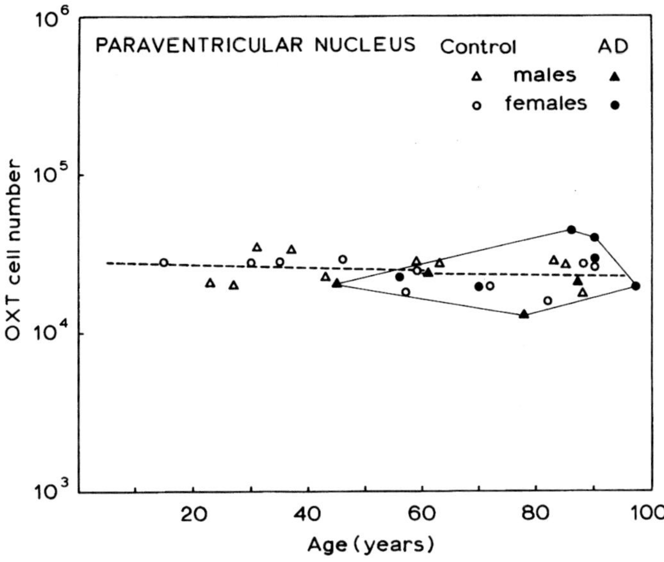

Fig. 2   Linear regression between OXT cell number in the PVN and age. Data of male and female control patients did not differ and were pooled. No statistically significant correlations were observed in either young or old control subjects. Values of male and female AD patients are delineated by a minimum convex polygon and were within the range of the controls. (From Wierda et al., 1991, with permission.)

number was observed (Fig. 2) [21, 18, 74, 70]. The observation that no cytoskeletal alterations were found in Alzheimer patients with several anti-bodies in the SON [64] is in accordance with this stability. Although in the PVN of Alzheimer patients some neuronal and dystrophic neurite staining is observed with cytoskeletal antibodies [64], the cell number in the PVN remains the same. Various observations provide evidence for the hypothesis that activation of neurons may interfere with the process of aging, and thus prolong the lifespan of neurons or restore their function. This hypothesis is paraphrased as 'use it or lose it' [63]. The SON and PVN neurons are not only metabolically highly active throughout life, but are extra activated in senescence as well, as can be judged from the increase in the size of the vasopressin-containing perikarya [13], nucleoli [23] and Golgi apparatus [35], and the enhanced plasma levels of vasopressin (Frolkis et al., 1982) and neurophysins [34]. Similar activation of vasopressin neurons was observed in the aged rat [12, 17] and is probably due to a loss of vasopressin receptors in the kidneys during aging [45].

In contrast to the SON, the PVN does not only contain magnocellular vasopressin and oxytocin neurons, but also parvicellular ones that project to central brain regions (see above) or to the median eminence. Examples of the latter type of neurons are the corticotropin-releasing hormone (CRH) neurons. In the human PVN they are not located in a well-defined subnucleus as they are in the rat, but are spread all over the PVN, except for the most rostral part where they are absent. Another property of CRH neurons in the PVN is that they co-express vasopressin when activated, as occurs in the process of aging [43].

4 Infundibular nucleus (arcuate nucleus)

The horseshoe-shaped infundibular (or arcuate) nucleus surrounds the lateral and posterior entrance of the infundibulum. It contains catecholamine-containing neurons [55], somatostatin, neuropeptide and neurotensin [52]. In 1966 Sheehan and Kovacs described neuronal hypertrophy in a sub-division of this nucleus in post-menopausal women and women suffering from postpartum hypopituitarism. Nucleolar size increase and multiplication confirm the activation of neurons in this area [68, 44]. This subdivision was named the **subventricular nucleus**, referring to its location; it is situated below and lateral to the third ventricle, and caudally to the tubero-infundibular sulcus. Infundibular neuronal hypertrophy has also been described in chronically ill, hypogonadal men and in patients suffering from starvation and gonadal atrophy [67], (for review see [44]). The hypertrophied neurons contain increased amounts of neurokinin B (NKB), substance P and estrogen receptor transcripts. LHRH neurons are also found in this nucleus, but the hypertrophied neurons themselves do not contain this peptide. The NKB-containing neurons probably participate in the hypothalamic circuitry, which regulates estrogen negative feedback on gonadotropin release in humans by acting as an interneuron on the LHRH-containing cells. In addition, the NKB neurons may be involved in the initiation of menopausal flushes [44].

5 Lateral tuberal nucleus

The lateral tuberal nucleus (nucleus tuberalis lateralis, NTL) is present in humans and higher primates. Macroscopically, the presence of the NTL is revealed by the "lateral eminence on the ventral surface of the tuber cinerium" [33]. The neurotransmitter content of the NTL and the connections with other parts of the brain are as yet unknown, but receptors for corticotropin-releasing factor, somatostatin, muscarinic cholinergic receptors, benzodiazepin receptors and N-methyl-D-aspartate (NMDA) receptors have been localized in the NTL [32]. In adulthood the NTL contains some 60,000 neurons, whereas in Huntington's disease this number may be reduced to less than 10,000 (Fig. 3), and gliosis is found depending on the age at onset of the disease as well as the age at death

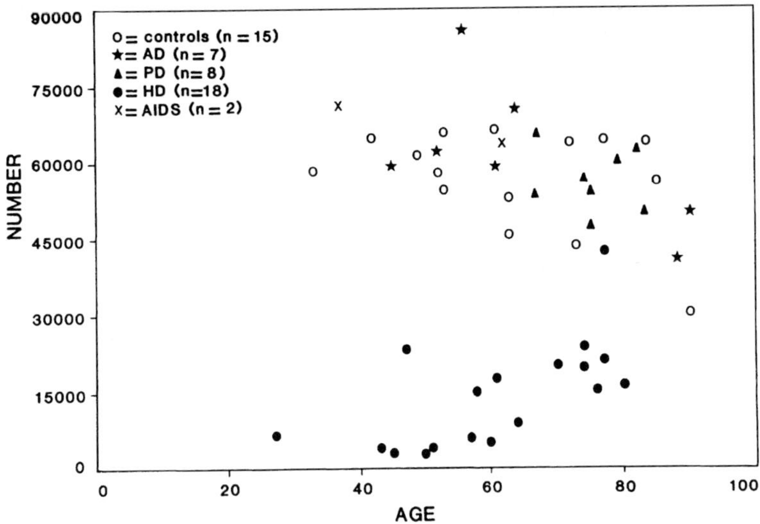

Fig. 3 Neuron number counts of the NTL in normal controls and neurological diseases. AD, Alzheimer's disease; PD, Parkinson's disease; HD, Huntington's disease; AIDS: acquired immunodeficiency syndrome. Linear regression analysis of neuronal numbers vs. age: for controls only (n = 15): neuron number = 71955 − (age 237.92), r = −0.38, P = 0.15; for the total group of controls, AD, PD and AIDS (n = 32): neuron number = 79126 − (age 315.19), r = −0.48, P = 0.0053. (From Kremer, 1992, with permission.)

[30]. Neuronal loss in the NTL may be a good marker of the severity of the disease, and the NTL may be one of the brain structures that is primarily affected by the Huntington's disease gene [32]. It is presumed that this NTL vulnerability is related to the high amount of NMDA receptors in this nucleus. Pathological changes in the NTL have also been described in depression [24], Kallman's syndrome [29] and dementia with intracranial argyrophilic grains and silver-staining coiled bodies containing straight filaments [4]. In Alzheimer's disease, the number of NTL neurons did not differ from that in controls. The number of plaques in this nucleus was low, and they were exclusively of the amorphous type. Neurofibrillary tangles were rare in conventional silver stainings. Yet immunocytochemical staining, using the monoclonal antibody Alz-50, showed such an abundant reactivity of both perikarya and neurites that the NTL of Alzheimer's disease patients could even be recognized by the naked eye [31]. Staining of Alzheimer hypothalami with anti-tau 1, anti-paired helical filaments and anti-ubiquitin showed about the same density of NTL neurons but far less neuritic staining [64]. The Alzheimer pattern of Alz-50 staining was also encountered in patients with Down's syndrome [32]. The NTL seems to represent a brain area in which Alzheimer's disease affects the neurons in a limited way, without further progress to the classical changes of silver-staining

of tangles and neuronal loss. Changes in Parkinson's disease are less obvious: Lewy bodies appear in small amounts, the majority of them apparently lying outside a neuronal perikaryan. No neuronal loss was found [32]. Lesions in the lateral hypothalamus of animals are known to be associated with weight loss. In Huntington's and in Alzheimer's disease dementia is combined with severe weight-loss in combination with normal or even increased food intake, as is the case in the condition described by Braak and Braak [4] and H. Braak (personal communication). Because NTL pathology is, in different conditions, accompanied by cachexia, the NTL is hypothesized to play a role in feeding behavior and metabolism. Animal experiments that are necessary to reveal such a role can only be performed when we can establish the homology between the NTL in human and a similar system in for example the rat. The observation (J. Van de Nes, unpubl. results) that somatostatin is a good marker of the NTL might be extremely helpful in this respect.

6 Tuberomammillary nucleus

The tuberomammillary nucleus (TM) is formed by large, irregularly bordered, darkly staining neurons that surround the NTL, the fornix in its final descending course, and the mammillary body [9]. Many of its neurons project extensively to the cortex [50]. For example, the major, if not the sole, histaminergic cortical innervation in rodents [56, 73] as well as in man [1, 41] originates from this group. For a long time now TM has been known to be affected by Alzheimer's disease: the occurrence of tangles and deposits of plaques can be found in this nucleus [26, 51, 54, 69). In the TM of Alzheimer patients we found numerous Alz-50 staining neurites. Neuritic staining with other cytoskeletal antibodies was markedly less than in NTL. In contrast to the NTL, the TM did show neurofibrillary tangles in Palmgren's silver impregnation [64]. In addition, Lewy body formation has been observed in the TM in Parkinson's disease [48]. Morphometrics have only been applied to a few subjects and concern Galanin neurons. Their number did not change in Alzheimer's or Parkinson's disease [6]. No clear qualitative changes in the number of histamine neurons were observed between Alzheimer patients and controls [6]. Although the NTL is seriously affected in Huntington's disease (see above) the surrounding neurons of the TM are not affected in this condition. Interestingly, contrary to the NTL, the TM does not contain NMDA receptors.

7 Summary and conclusions

The SCN coordinates circadian and circannual rhythms. A marked seasonal and circadian variation in the volume and vasopressin cell number of the SCN was observed in relation to the variation in photoperiod. During normal aging, the number of vasopressin neurons decreases. In Alzheimer's disease, the decrease in cell number is even more pronounced and cytoskeletal alterations are observed. This pathology might be the neural basis for the nightly restlessness observed in patients suffering from Alzheimer's disease, whereas degeneration of the visual system input to the SCN might contribute to these functional disturbances. It is exciting, therefore, to see that stimulation of the visual pathways by light therapy seems to improve the disturbances in behavior in Alzheimer patients.

Recently, we found that the SCN in homosexual men is about twice as large as that of a reference group. The functional meaning of this observation is not yet clear.

The SDN (intermediate nucleus or INAH-1) is localized between the supraoptic and paraventricular nucleus. In adult men the SDN is twice as large as in adult women. In girls, the SDN shows a decreasing cell number during pre-pubescent development, leading to sexual dimorphism. During aging a decrease in cell number is found in both sexes. The latter change may be related to a decrease in sexual activity and to changes in hormone levels. In Alzheimer's disease cytoskeletal changes are found in the SDN, but SDN cell numbers decrease at a similar rate as in normal aging. Since the SDN in homo- and heterosexual men is similar in size and cell number, the hypothesis that homosexual men have a female hypothalamus is not supported.

The cells of the SON and PVN produce vasopressin or oxytocin. These nuclei are examples of neuron populations that seem to stay perfectly intact in aging and Alzheimer's disease. The cells do not show cytoskeletal changes in Alzheimer's disease. We hypothesize that this might be due to the activation of these neuroendocrine cells during the aging process. On the other hand, in other conditions the PVN may be affected, since the oxytocin neuron number is 50% lower in Prader-Willi syndrome, 40% lower in AIDS and 20% lower in Parkinson's disease.

Parvicellular corticotropin-releasing hormone (CRH)-containing neurons are found throughout the PVN. CRH neurons are activated in the course of aging as appears from the increasing proportion of neurons showing co-localization with vasopressin.

The subventricular nucleus contains hypertrophic neurons in postmenopausal women, in hypogonadal men, and in conditions such as starvation and postpartum hypopituitarism. The hypertrophied neurons contain neurokinin-B (NKB), substance-P and estrogen receptors and probably act on LHRH neurons as interneurons. The NKB neurons may also be involved in the initiation of menopausal flushes.

The NTL and TM are lateral structures of the tuberal region. The NTL might be involved in feeding behavior and metabolism. In Huntington's disease the majority of NTL neurons are lost. Although it does not show any decrease in neuronal numbers in Alzheimer's disease, a very strong Alz-50 staining is present in the NTL of Alzheimer patients, which is due to a dense network of dystrophic neurites and numerous staining perikarya. The NTL in Alzheimer's disease patients seems, therefore, to be in an early phase of the disease process. In addition, we may conclude that Alz-50 is not simply a marker for impending cell death. In Parkinson's disease only a few Lewy bodies are found, and no cell loss is observed.

Tuberomammillary nucleus (TM) neurons project to the cortex. Neurons contain histamine or galanin. Their number does not seem to diminish in Alzheimer's disease, although TM neurons show cytoskeletal alterations, plaques and tangles. In addition, Lewy bodies have been observed in the TM of Parkinson patients.

It can be concluded that the various hypothalamic nuclei are involved in a great number of functions and show clear and differential changes in development with respect to sex, in menopause, in aging and in a number of neurological diseases. We believe that only a small proportion of such changes have, at present, been identified.

Acknowledgements

Brain material was obtained from the Netherlands Brain Bank, Amsterdam (coordinator Dr. R. Ravid). The authors would like to express their thanks to Ms. W. Verweij for her secretarial help, and Mr. G. Van der Meulen for his photographic work. As part of the AMSTEL project, part of this study was supported by the Stimuleringsprogramma Gezondheidsonderzoek (SGO) of the Netherlands Ministry of Science and Education. Financial support was also obtained from Mrs. E. J. M. Stevens.

References

[1] Airaksinen, M. S., A. Paer, L. Paljärvi et al.: Histamine neurons in human hypothalamus: anatomy in normal and Alzheimer diseased brains. Neurosci. **44** (1991) 465−481.

[2] Allen, L. S., M. Hines, J. E. Shryne et al.: Sex difference in the bed nucleus of the stria terminalis of the human brain. J. Comp. Neurol. **302** (1989) 697−706.

[3] Braak, H., E. Braak: The hypothalamus of the human adult: chiasmatic region. Anat. Embryol. **176** (1987) 315−330.

[4] Braak, H., E. Braak: Cortical and subcortical argyrophylic grains characterize a disease associated with adult onset dementia. Neuropathol. Appl. Neurobiol. 15 (1989) 13−26.

[5] Campbell, S. S., D. F. Kripke, J. C. Gillin et al.: Exposure to light in healthy elderly subjects and Alzheimer patients. Physiol. Behav. 42 (1988) 141−144.

[6] Chan-Palay, V. L., B. Jentsch: Galinin tuberomammillary neurons in the hypothalamus in Alzheimer's and Parkinson's disease. In: D. F. Swaab, M. A. Hofman, M. Mirmiran et al. (eds.): The Human Hypothalamus in Health and Disease. Progress in Brain Research vol. 93, pp. 263−270, Elsevier, Amsterdam 1992.

[7] Cohen, R. A. and H. E. Albers: Disruption of human circadian and cognitive regulation following a discrete hypothalamic lesion: a case study. Neurology 41 (1991) 726−729.

[8] De Jonge, F. H., A. L. Louwerse, M. P. Ooms et al.: Lesions of the SDN-POA inhibit sexual behaviour of male Wistar rats. Brain Res. Bull. 23 (1989) 483−492.

[9] Diepen, R.: Der Hypothalamus. In: W. Bargmann (ed.) Handbuch der mikroskopischen Anatomie des Menschen IV/7, pp. 1−181, Springer, Berlin 1962.

[10] Dörner, G.: Neuroendocrine response to estrogen and brain differentiation in heterosexuals, homosexuals, and transsexuals. Arch. Sexual Behav. 17 (1988) 57−75.

[11] Fekete, M., J. M. Van Ree, R. J. M. Niesink et al.: Disruption of circadian rhythms induces retrograde amnesia. Physiol. Behav. 34 (1985) 883−887.

[12] Fliers, E., D. F. Swaab: Activation of vasopressinergic and oxytocinergic neurons during aging in the Wistar rat. Peptides 4 (1983) 165−170.

[13] Fliers, E., G. J. De Vries, D. F. Swaab: Changes with aging in the vasopressin and oxytocin innervation of the rat brain. Brain Res. 348 (1985) 1−8.

[14] Fliers, E., S. E. F. Guldenaar, N. Van de Wal et al.: Extrahypothalamic vasopressin and oxytocin in the human brain; presence of vasopressin cells in the bed nucleus of the stria terminalis. Brain Res. 375 (1986) 363−367.

[15] Gladue, B. A., R. Green, R. E. Helleman: Neuroendocrine response to estrogen and sexual orientation. Science 225 (1984) 1496−1499.

[16] Gorski, R. A., J. H. Gordon, J. E. Shryne: Evidence for a morphological sex difference whithin the medial preoptic area of the rat brain. Brain Res. 148 (1978) 333−346.

[17] Goudsmit, E., E. Fliers, D. F. Swaab: Vasopressin and oxytocin excretion in the Brown Norway rat in relation to aging, water metabolism and testosterone. Mech. of Ageing and Development 44 (1988) 241−252.

[18] Goudsmit, E., M. A. Hofman, E. Fliers et al.: The supraoptic and paraventricular nuclei of the human hypothalamus in relation to sex, age and Alzheimer's disease. Neurobiol. Aging 11 (1990) 529−536.

[19] Hinton, D. R., A. A. Sadun, J. C. Blanks et al.: Optic nerve degeneration in Alzheimer's disease. N. Engl. J. Med. 315 (1986) 485−487.

[20] Hofman, M. A., D. F. Swaab: The sexually dimorphic nucleus of the preoptic area in the human brain: a comparative morphometric study. J. Anat. 164 (1989) 55−72.

[21] Hofman, M. A., E. Goudsmit, J. S. Purba et al.: Morphometric analysis of the supraoptic nucleus in the human brain. J. Anat. 172 (1990) 259−270.

[22] Hofman, M. A., D. F. Swaab: Seasonal changes in the suprachiasmatic nucleus of man. Neurosci. Lett. 139 (1992) 257−260.

[23] Hoogendijk, J. E., E. Fliers, D. F. Swaab et al.: Activation of vasopressin neurons in the human supraoptic and paraventricular nucleus in senescence and senile dementia. J. Neurol. Sci. 69 (1985) 291−299.

[24] Horn, E., B. Lach, Y. Lapierre et al.: Hypothalamic pathology in the neuroleptic malignant syndrome. Am. J. Psychiatry 145 (1988) 617−620.

[25] Insel, T. R.: Oxytocin − a neuropeptide for affiliation: evidence from behavioral, receptor autoradiographic, and comparative studies. Psychoneuroendocrinology 17 (1992) 3−35.

[26] Ishii, T.: Distribution of Alzheimer's neurofibrillary changes in the brain stem and hypothalamus of senile dementia. Acta Heuropathol. **6** (1966) 181–187.

[27] Jacobson, C. D., J. E. Shryne, F. Shapiro et al.: Ontogeny of the sexually dimorphic nucleus of the preoptic area. J. Comp. Neurol. **193** (1980) 541–548.

[28] Katz, B., S. Rimmer, V. Iragui et al.: Abnormal pattern electroretinogram in Alzheimer's disease: evidence for retinal ganglion cell degeneration? Ann. Neurol. **26** (1989) 221–225.

[29] Kovacs, K., H. L. Sheehan: Pituitary changes in Kallman's syndrome. A histologic, immunocytologic, ultrastructural, and immunoelectron microscopic study. Fert. Steril. **37** (1982) 83–89.

[30] Kremer, H. P. H., R. A. C. Roos, G. Dingjan et al.: Atrophy of the hypothalamic lateral tuberal nucleus in Huntington's disease. J. Neuropathol. Exp. Neurol. **49** (1990) 371–382.

[31] Kremer, H. P. H., D. F. Swaab, G. Th. A. M. Bots et al.: The hypothalamic lateral tuberal nucleus in Alzheimer's disease. Ann. Neurol. **29** (1991) 279–284.

[32] Kremer, H. P. H.: The hypothalamic lateral tuberal nucleus: normal anatomy and changes in neurological diseases. In: D. F. Swaab, M. A. Hofman, M. Mirmiran et al. (eds.): The Human Hypothalamus in Health and Disease, Progress in Brain Research vol. 93, pp. 249–261, Elsevier, Amsterdam 1992.

[33] Le Gros Clark, W. E.: Morphological aspects of the hypothalamus. In: W. E. Le Gros Clark, J. Beattie, G. Riddoch et al. (eds.) The Hypothalamus. Morphological, Functional, Clinical and Surgical Aspects, pp. 1–68, Oliver and Boyd, Edinburgh 1938.

[34] Legros, J. J., P. Gilot, S. Schmitz et al.: Neurohypophyseal peptides and cognitive function: a clinical approach. In: F. Brambilla, G. Racagni, D. de Wied (eds.) Progress in Psychoneuroendocrinology, pp. 325–337, Elsevier Science Publishers, Amsterdam 1980.

[35] Lucassen, P. J., D. F. Swaab, R. Ravid et al.: Activation of the Golgi-apparatus in human supraoptic and paraventricular neurons with aging and in Alzheimer's disease (1993, in prep.).

[36] Mai, J. K., O. Kedziora, L. Teckhaus et al.: Evidence for subdivisions in the human suprachiasmatic nucleus. J. Comp. Neurol. **305** (1991) 508–525.

[37] Mirmiran, M., J. Overdijk, W. Witting et al.: A simple method for recording and analyzing circadian rhythms in man. J. Neurosci. Meth. **25** (1988) 209–214.

[38] Moore, R. Y.: The organization of the human circadian timing system. In: D. F. Swaab, M. A. Hofman, M. Mirmiran et al. (eds.) The Human Hypothalamus in Health and Disease, Progress in Brain Research vol. 93, pp. 99–117, Elsevier, Amsterdam 1992.

[39] Murphy, M. R., J. R. Seckl, S. Burton et al.: Changes in oxytocin and vasopressin secretion during sexual activity in men. J. Clin. Endocrin. Metab. **65** (1987) 738–741.

[40] Okawa, M., Y. Hishikawa, S. Hozumi et al.: Sleep-wake rhythm disorder and phototherapy in elderly patients with dementia. In: G. Racagni et al. (eds.) Biological Psychiatry 1 (1991) 837–840.

[41] Panula, P., M. S. Airaksinen, U. Pirvola et al.: Histamine containing neuronal system in human brain. Neuroscience **34** (1990) 129–132.

[42] Prinz, P. N., P. P. Viatliano, M. V. Vitiello et al.: Sleep, EEG and mental function changes in senile sementia of the Alzheimer's type. Neurobiol. Aging **3** (1982) 361–370.

[43] Raadsheer, F. C., A. A. Sluiter, R. Ravid et al.: Localization of corticotropin-releasing hormone (CRH) neurons in the paraventricular nucleus of the human hypothalamus; age-dependent colocalization with vasopressin. **615** (1993, pp. 50–62).

[44] Rance, N. E.: Hormonal influences on morphology and neuropeptide gene expression in the infundibular nucleus of post-menopausal women. In: D. F. Swaab, M. A. Hofman, M. Mirmiran et al. (eds.) The Human Hypothalamus in Health and Disease, Progress in Brain Research vol. 93, pp. 221–236, Elsevier, Amsterdam 1992.

[45] Ravid, R., E. Fliers, D. F. Swaab et al.: Changes in vasopressin and testosterone in the senescent Brown-Norway (BN/BiRij) rat. Gerontology **33** (1987) 87–98.

[46] Rusak, B., I. Zucker: Neural regulation of circadian rhythms. Physiol. Rev. **59** (1979) 449–526.

[47] Sack, R. L., A. J. Lewy, M. L. Blood et al.: Circadian Rhythm Abnormalities in totally blind people: incidence and clinical significance. J. Clin. Endocrin. Metab. **75** (1992) 127–134.

[48] Sandyk, R., R. P. Iacono, C. R. Bamford: The hypothalamus in Parkinson's disease. Ital. J. Neurol. Sci. 8(3) (1987) 227–234.

[49] Sanford, J. R. A.: Tolerance of debility in elderly dependents by supporters at home: its significance for hospital practice. Br. Med. J. 3 (1975) 471–473.

[50] Saper, C. B.: Organization of cerebral cortical afferent systems in the rat. II Hypothalamocortical projections. J. Comp. Neurol. **237** (1985) 21–46.

[51] Saper, C. B., D. C. German: Hypothalamic pathology in Alzheimer's disease. Neurosci. Lett. **74** (1987) 364–370.

[52] Saper, C. B.: Hypothalamus. In: G. Paxinos (ed.): The Human Nervous System, pp. 389–413, Academic Press, San Diego 1990.

[53] Schwartz, W. J., N. A. Bosis, E. T. Hedley-Whyte: A discrete lesion of ventral hypothalamus and optic chiasm that disturbed the daily temperature rhythm. J. Neurol. **233** (1986) 1–4.

[54] Simpson, W. A., C. M. Yates, A. G. Watts et al.: Congo red birefringent structures in the hypothalamus in senile dementia of the Alzheimer type. Neuropathol. Appl. Neurobiol. **14** (1988) 381–393.

[55] Spencer, S., C. B. Saper, T. Joh et al.: Distribution of catecholamine-containing neurons in the normal human hypothalamus. Brain Res. *328* (1985) 73–80.

[56] Steinbusch, H. W. M., A. H. Mulder: Localization and projections of histamine immunoreactive neurons in the central nervous system of the rat. In: A. Björklund, T. Hökfelt, M. J. Kuhar (eds.): Handbook of Chemical Neuroanatomy 3, pp. 126–140, Elsevier, Amsterdam 1984.

[57] Swaab, D. F., E. Fliers: A sexually dimorphic nucleus in the human brain. Science **228** (1985) 1112–1115.

[58] Swaab, D. F., E. Fliers, T. S. Partiman: The suprachiasmatic nucleus of the human brain in relation to sex, age and senile dementia. Brain Res. **342** (1985) 37–44.

[59] Swaab, D. F., B. Roozendaal, R. Ravid: Suprachiasmatic nucleus in aging, Alzheimer's disease, transsexuality and Prader-Willi syndrome. In: E. R. De Kloet, V. M. Wiegant, D. De Wied (eds.): Neuropeptides and Brain Function, Progress in Brain Research vol. 72, pp. 301–310, Elsevier, Amsterdam 1987.

[60] Swaab, D. F., M. A. Hofman: Sexual differentiation of the human hypothalamus: ontogeny of the sexually dimorphic nucleus of the preoptic area. Dev. Brain Res. **44** (1988) 314–318.

[61] Swaab, D. F., M. A. Hofman, M. B. O. M. Honnebier: Development of vasopressin neurons in the human suprachiasmatic nucleus in relation to birth. Dev. Brain Res. **52** (1990) 289–293.

[62] Swaab, D. F., M. A. Hofman: An enlarged suprachiasmatic nucleus in homosexual men. Brain Res. **537** (1990) 141–148.

[63] Swaab, D. F.: Brain aging and Alzheimer's disease: "wear and tear" versus "use it or lose it". Neurobiol. Aging **12** (1991) 317–324.

[64] Swaab, D. F., I. Grundke-Iqbal, K. Iqbal et al.: Tau and ubiquitin in the human hypothalamus in aging and Alzheimer's disease. Brain Res. **590** [1992] 239–249.

[65] Trick, G. L., M. C. Barris, M. Bickler-Bluth: Abnormal pattern electroretinograms in patients with senile dementia of the Alzeimer type. Ann. Neurol. **26** (1989) 226–231.

[66] Turkenburg, J. L., D. F. Swaab, E. Endert et al.: Effects of lesions of the sexually dimorphic nucleus on sexual behaviour of testosterone-treated female Wistar rats. Brain Res. Bull. **21** (1988) 215–224.

[67] Ule, G., C. Walter: Morphological feedback effect on the nucleoli of the neurons in the nucleus arcuatus (infundibularis) to hypophyseal hypogonadism in juvenile haemochromatosis. Acta Neuropathol. **61** (1983) 81–84.

[68] Ule, G., K. Schwechheimer, C. Tschahargane: Morphological feedback effect on neurons of the nucl. arcuatus (sive infundibularis) and nucl. subventricularis hypothalami due to gonadal atrophy. Virchows Arch. 400 (1983) 297–308.

[69] Ulfig, N., H. Braak: Amyloid deposits and neurofibrillary changes in the hypothalamic tubero-mammillary nucleus. J. Neural. Transm. (P. D. Sect) 1 (1984) 143.

[70] Van der Woude, P. F., E. Goudsmit, M. Wierda et al.: Increase in the number of vasopressin immunoreactive cells in the human paraventricular nucleus with normal aging, but not in Alzheimer's disease (1993, in prep.).

[71] Van Gool, W. A., M. Mirmiran: Aging and circadian rhythms. In: Swaab, D. F. et al. (eds.) Aging of the Brain and Alzheimer's Disease, Progress in Brain Research vol. 70, pp. 255–279, Elsevier, Amsterdam 1986.

[72] Vermeulen, A.: Androgens and male senescence. In: E. Nieschlag, H. M. Behre (eds.) Testosterone, Action Deficiency Substitution. pp. 261–276, Springer Verlag, Berlin 1990.

[73] Watanabe, T., Y. Taguchi, S. Shiosaka et al.: Distribution of the histaminergic neuron system in the central nervous system of rats: a fluorescent immunohistochemical analysis with histidine decarboxylase as a marker. Brain Res. 295 (1984) 13–25.

[74] Wierda, M., E. Goudsmit, P. F. Van der Woude et al.: Oxytocin cell number in the human paraventricular nucleus remains constant with aging and in Alzheimer's disease. Neurobiol. Aging 12 (1991) 511–516.

[75] Witting, W., I. H. Kwa, P. Eikelenboom et al.: Alterations in the circadian rest-activity rhythm in aging and Alzheimer's disease. Biol. Psychiatry 27 (1990) 563–572.

Age-related changes in psychoneuroendocrinological function

I. Heuser

The hypothalamic-pituitary-adrenal (HPA) system is one of the major endocrine systems to regulate stress-adaptive mechanisms so that homeostasis is maintained whenever the organism's "balance" is challenged. The HPA system and its key hormones corticotropin-releasing hormone (CRH), adreno-corticotropin (ACTH) and glucocorticoids, are regulated by a variety of neurotransmitters and other hormonal systems and, in turn, stimulate or inhibit synthesis and/or release of neurotransmitters and hormones (Fig. 1) [10].

Activation of the HPA system as a response to cognitive (e. g., perception) and non-cognitive (e. g., infection) stressors ultimately results in an increased glucocorticoid secretion from the adrenals, which leads to numerous metabolic changes in order to prepare the organism for an adequate response ("fight or flight").

As indicated in Fig. 1, adrenal corticosteroids feed back negatively to the hippocampus, hypothalamus and anterior pituitary to restrain excessive adreno-cortical activation. Concerted genomic and non-genomic effects of adrenal steroids result in three distinguishable time schemes of negative feedback action:

1. Fast feedback (up to 10 minutes), affecting the release of CRH, vasopressin (AVP) and other ACTH secretagogues from the median eminence;
2. intermediate feedback (up to 1 to 2 hours), involving steroid effects on stimulus-secretion-coupling, excitability and intracellular signal transduction pathways; and
3. slow-feedback (several hours), regulating suppression of stress-induced CRH- and AVP-gene expression in the parvocellular neurons of the nucleus paraventricularis (PVN) and proopio-melanocortin (POMC)-gene expression in corticotrophic cells.

Recent research in animals has demonstrated that the negative feedback machinery at the hippocampal level preserves its flexibility by using a binary cortico-steroid receptor system: 1. the mineralocortico-steroid receptor (MR) and 2. the glucocorticoid receptor (GR) [3]. While GRs are rather ubiquitously distributed throughout the brain, MRs predominate in the hippocampus. Both types of these hippocampal receptors bind glucocorticoids, but the MR with a 6- to 10-fold higher affinity than the GR. While MR occupancy varies between

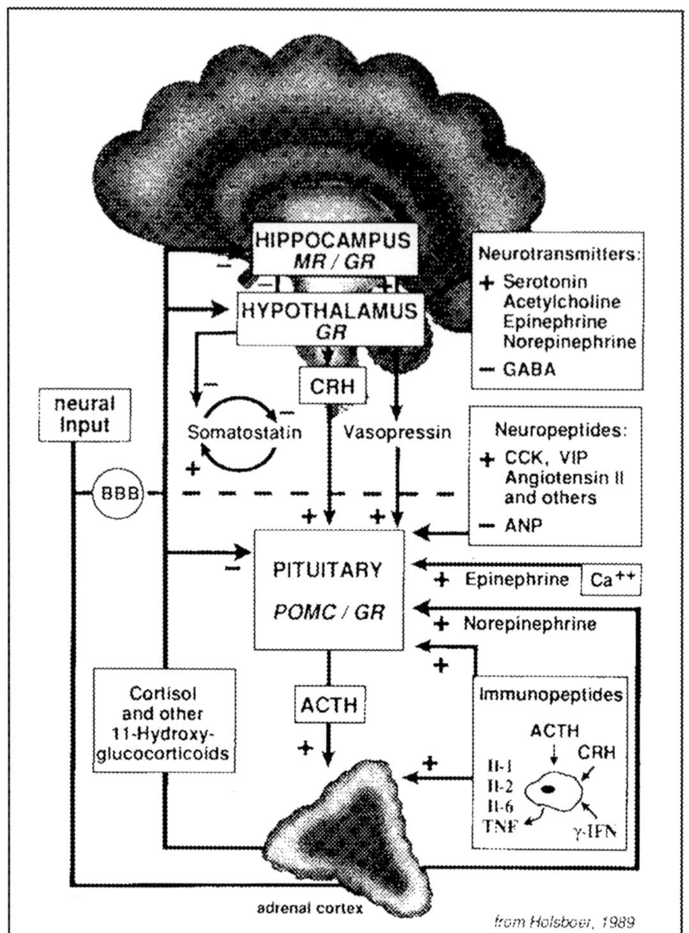

Fig. 1   Hypothalamic-pituitary-adrenal (HPA) system.

MR	=	Mineralocorticoid-Receptor	ANP	=	Atrial Naturetic Peptide
GR	=	Glucocorticoid-Receptor	BBB	=	Blood-Brain-Barrier
CRH	=	Corticotropin-Releasing Hormone	ACTH	=	Corticotropin
CCK	=	Cholecystokinin	IFN-γ	=	Interferon-gamma
VIP	=	Vasointestinal Peptide	IL1, 2, 6	=	Interleukine 1, 2, 6
			TNF	=	Tumor-Necrosis-Factor

70% and 90%, that of GR varies from 10% to 90%, depending on levels of circulating glucocorticoids; thus, steroid-binding of MR varies over a much lower range than that of GR. Occupation of hippocampal MR maintains tonic inhibitory control over the HPA system, whereas GR activation, for example induced by higher levels of glucocorticoids during stress or circadian surges, opposes this MR effect (for review: [11]).

The neuroendocrine system plays a major role in controlling certain aging processes and may be involved in the development of pathology, which becomes more likely with increasing age. Studies in aged rats showed increased circulating basal levels of glucocorticoids, impaired adrenocortical recovery from stress and a substantial neuronal loss in the hippocampal formation [19, 20]. To date, it still remains to be elucidated which component of the HPA system contributes to age-related HPA overdrive: it is speculated that, with aging, an increased basal and stress-responsive hypothalamic CRH activity occurs and/or changes in pituitary glucocorticoid and CRH-receptor number/density and possibly an age-related increase in adrenal sensitivity to ACTH develop.

It is assumed that repeated "stressful" life events − as they inevitably occur during an individual's life − paralleled by markedly increased glucocorticoid secretion, ultimately compromise the hippocampus' buffering capacity upon glucocorticoid regulation. This line of reasoning is supported by the fact that neuropathological studies in humans have shown degenerative changes in hippocampal neurons as early as the fourth decade of life [2]. Further, the neurons of layers CA_3 are highly vulnerable to altered brain metabolism, such as hypoxia and hypoglycemia, events − ever so subtle − that are most likely to take place in advanced age [20].

There is considerable evidence from animal studies of an age-associated reduction in the number of corticosteroid receptors in the hippocampus [13, 16]. These age-associated neuronal changes would imply that, with aging, the HPA system becomes progressively more disinhibited, "peripherally" reflected by basal hypercortisolemia and an increased glucocorticoid response to an acute or chronic stressor. Several studies in humans and animals do support the notion that such a cascade of events ("cascade theory") occurs with aging [26, 21, 18]. However, the cascade theory has not remained undisputed: the concept of a binary glucocorticoid receptor system, as elaborated by de Kloet and co-workers, which regulates glucocorticoid feedback via hippocampal MR and GR, assumes that age-associated adaptive changes in central MR- and GR-mediated effects take place, which consequently alter the setpoint of homeostatic control ("balance theory"; for review: [3]). Such a model offers some explanation why in several studies no age-related changes in basal and stimulus-induced glucocorticoid secretion were observable, despite the finding of decreased hippocampal glucocorticoid receptor (MR and GR) numbers in old animals [23].

Results from studies in human aging, addressing changes in cortisol secretion and in feedback regulation, yield ambiguous results: increases in the percentage of cortisol non-suppression after dexamethasone and higher basal cortisol concentrations were found in the elderly [15, 5, 4]. However, other studies in humans report no difference in HPA-system regulation between young and old subjects [14, 28, 1, 17, 27], and one study reported even **lower** 24-hour cortisol plasma concentrations in elderly (66−89 years) compared to young subjects (19−25 years) [22].

Patients with depression or other psychiatric disorders frequently have symptom clusters (sleep disturbances, altered eating behavior, decreased libido, cardiovascular changes, cognitive deficits and changes in hormone secretion) which strongly point to involvement of the HPA system as a relay station between neurocircuitries in the brain and peripheral hormone and autonomic nervous function.

Approximately 50%−60% of patients with a major depressive disorder are hypercortisolemic and, frequently, they escape cortisol suppression after dexamethasone (dexamethasone suppression test; DST). Further, it was shown that depressed patients had a blunted ACTH response after i.v. administration of a test dose of CRH (CRH test), and that the amount of ACTH produced and

23.00 h (previous night): 1.5 mg dexamethasone orally

12.00 h	lunch
13.30 h	i.v. started ("through the wall")
14.00-15.00 h	blood sampling every 15 minutes
15.00 h	100µg hCRH i.v.
15.00-18.00 h	blood sampling every 15 minutes

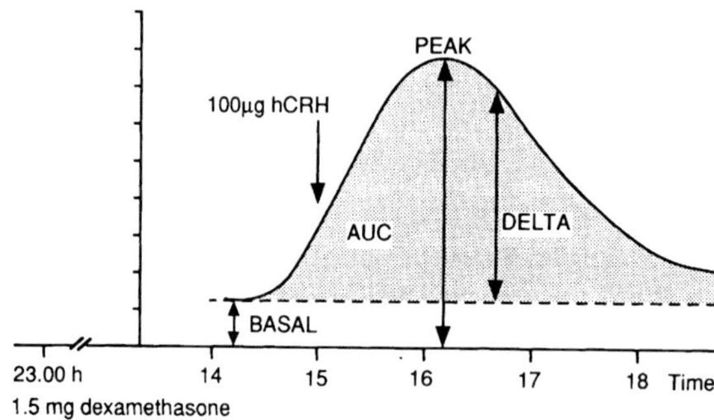

Fig. 2   Combined dexamethasone suppression/CRH-stimulation (DEX/CRH) test.
BASAL   = mean hormone secretion between 1400 and 1500 h (after dexamethasone, but prior to CRH)
PEAK   = maximum between 1500 and 1800 h (after additional CRH injection)
DELTA   = maximum between 1500 and 1800 h (after additional CRH injection) corrected for BASAL secretion
AUC   = area under the curve between 1500 and 1800 h (after additional CRH injection) corrected for BASAL secretion

released after CRH stimulation was inversely related to basal cortisol secretion. It was further observed that the cortisol response after CRH among depressives was indistinguishable from those of controls, despite significantly lower ACTH release in the former subjects. This points to a hypersensitive adrenal cortex, resulting from long-term overexposure to ACTH, confirming conclusions drawn from ACTH and cortisol profiles at baseline and after ACTH challenges (for review: [9]). Furthermore, pretreatment of depressives with metyrapone, which suppresses cortisol biosynthesis, was found to result in normalized ACTH release after CRH stimulation [25]. From these data, it was concluded that elevated circulating cortisol was the main, but not sole, abnormality preventing adequate ACTH response via negative feedback. In addition to basal hypercortisolism, other mechanisms, which might account for blunted ACTH responses to CRH in depressed patients, must be considered (e. g., altered processing and/or storage of ACTH precursors; desensitized CRH receptors at the pituitary corticotrophs; alternative processing of POMC molecules).

In normal controls, increasing dosages of dexamethasone result in a dose-dependent decrease of the measurable amount of ACTH secreted after subsequent human CRH stimulation. Our group was the first to combine the dexamethasone-suppression test (DST) and the CRH-challenge test in what was named the "combined dexamethasone-suppression CRH-stimulation (DEX/CRH) test" ([24] Fig. 2). The hypothesis was that, due to the elevated levels of endogenous corticosteroids frequently found in depressed patients, even lower dexamethasone dosages would suffice to prevent further ACTH release following CRH. Contrary to expectation the opposite was found (Fig. 3): In depressed

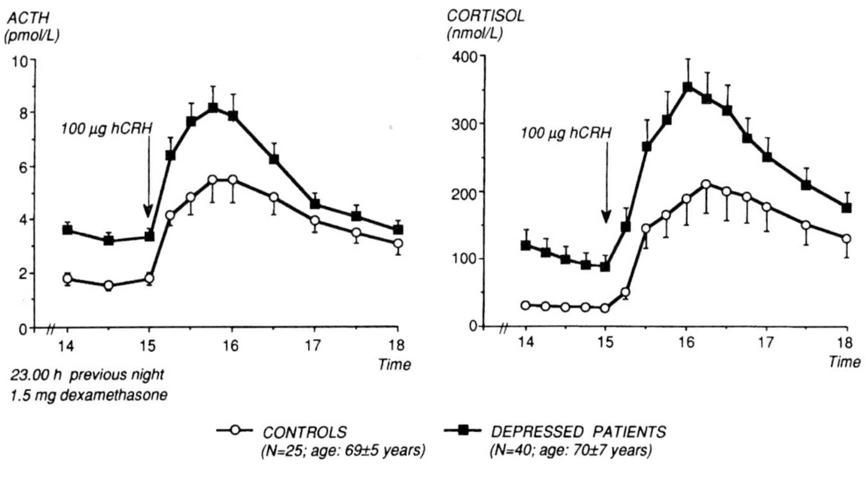

Fig. 3 DEX/CRH-test results in depressed patients and control subjects (data are presented as means ± SEM).

patients, dexamethasone (DEX) pretreatment did not suppress, but enhance, the pituitary responsiveness to CRH [24]. This exaggerated cortisol and ACTH response after DEX and additional CRH administration proved to be a state-dependent phenomenon, mimicking endocrinologically the clinical course of the individual patient [12, 7]. The explanation for this paradoxical phenomenon might be as follows: repeated phasic activation of the HPA system, as it occurs during chronic stress conditions (e. g., psychiatric illness, physical activity), might uncover an underlying, yet under resting conditions (dormant) positive feedback mechanism of glucocorticoids, which overrides the normally negative feedback regulation of steroid secretion. However, the underlying mechanisms of these seemingly paradoxical feedback "switches" unveiled by CRH challenge under DEX-pretreatment conditions remain unclear.

In a study by our group, we measured baseline secretion of ACTH and cortisol in 10 young (< 30 years) and 10 old (> 60 years) healthy volunteers every 15 minutes, from 1400 to 2000 h. At 1700 h, these individuals were subjected to a computerized cognitive challenge test, lasting 45 minutes. The results of this study indicate that there is no difference in baseline, pre-stress spontaneous hormone secretion (1400−1700 h) between young and old controls. However, the older subjects had significantly higher cortisol responses to the mental challenge test than the younger volunteers (Fig. 4). Further, 40 (22 males, 18 females) elderly (69 ± 5 years) and 20 young (34 ± 8 years; 15 males, 5 females) volunteers underwent a DEX/CRH test, as described above. Results revealed that the DEX-pretreated, "basal" (1400−1500 h) ACTH concentration was not

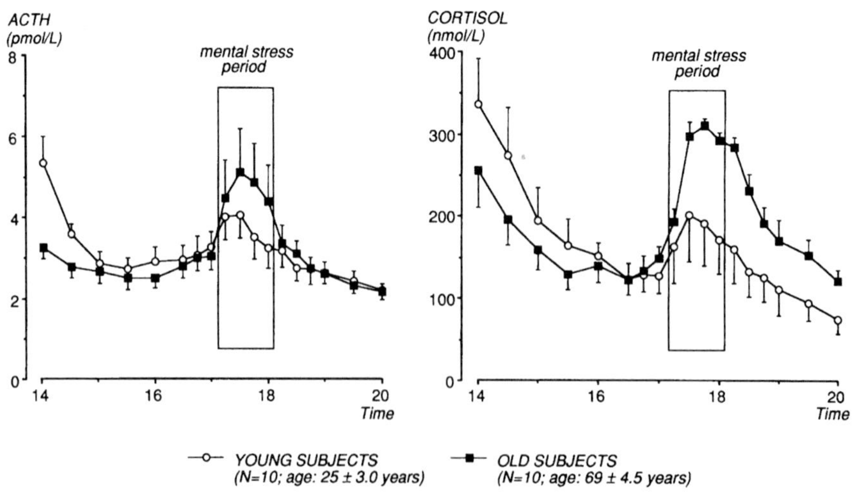

Fig. 4 ACTH and cortisol baseline secretion and hormonal response to a mental stress in young versus old subjects (data are presented as means ± SEM).

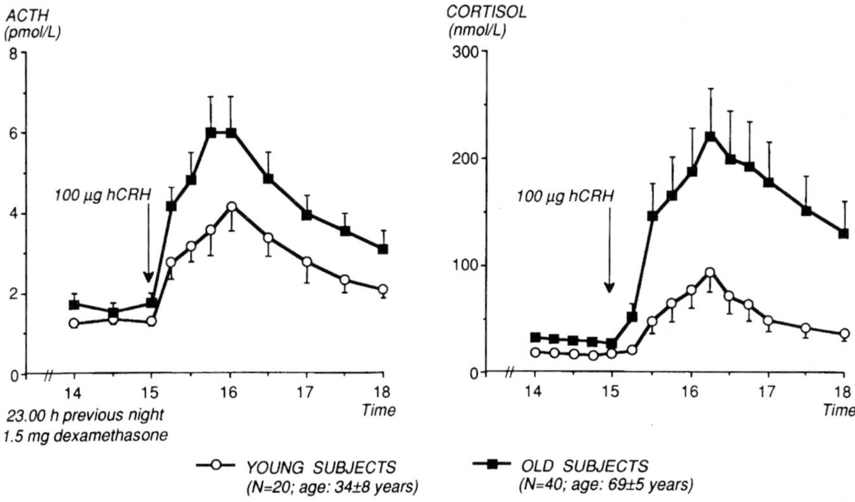

Fig. 5   DEX/CRH-test results in young and old subjects (data are presented as means ± SEM).

different between older and younger subjects, whereas the former had statistically significantly higher "basal" cortisol levels in comparison to their younger counterparts (Fig. 5). However, none of the subjects studied, regardless of age, escaped cortisol suppression after DEX **and** before subsequent CRH administration, none got even close to the critical cutoff point of 110 nmol/L cortisol for DST non-suppression. Only 25% (5/20) of the young controls exceeded the critical mark of 110 nmol/L cortisol **after** additional CRH bolus injection, as opposed to 53% (21/40) of the old subjects [6]. These data show that age profoundly affects HPA-system functioning in healthy humans, a fact which would have gone unnoticed if only measurement of spontaneous (1400–1700 h hormone profiles) hormone secretion or the "standard DST" had been employed. Since all volunteers in our study, regardless of age, showed normal suppression of cortisol and ACTH after DEX and **before** CRH, the suggestion is that the unchallenged HPA system of older individuals is capable of maintaining overt cortisol homeostasis and that subtle changes become evident only if more sophisticated challenge paradigms are used (DEX/CRH test); mental stress paradigm). This notion is also corroborated by our finding of unaltered spontaneous hormone secretion in older subjects, despite a much more profound cortisol release as response to a mental challenge test.

The assumption that a greater frequency of episodes with glucocorticoid excess results in an acquired insensitivity of the glucocorticoid feedback signal is further substantiated by our previously reported finding in elderly marathon runners, who were found to have increased cortisol and ACTH responses to CRH after dexamethasone pretreatment in comparison to age-matched sedentary controls, and similar, albeit different from depressed age-matched patients, suppressed cortisol concentrations after DEX and before CRH [8].

From the above-mentioned studies in humans it is concluded that, during aging, hippocampal neurons gradually become defunct. This deficit, however, can be transiently buffered by adaptive changes in the ratio of MR and GR, enabling the organism to maintain regular, basal cortisol levels and adequately suppressed cortisol after DEX as well as after DEX **and** subsequent CRH administration. With time, however, an acquired hippocampal insensitivity to rapidly rising cortisol levels may develop but may only become apparent in a paradigm, such as the DEX/CRH test or the mental challenge test. It might very well be that, in very old age, spontaneous hypercortisolemia in humans may finally occur, meaning that "balance" is no longer maintained but a "cascade" of events takes place, ultimately resulting in a vicious circle.

References

[1] Ansseau, M., R. von Frenckell, C. Simon et al.: Prediction of cortisol response to dexamethasone from age and basal cortisol in normal volunteers: A negative study. Psychopharmacology **90** (1986) 276−277.

[2] Ball, M. J.: Neuronal loss, neurofibrillary tangles and granulovacuolar degeneration in the hippocampus with aging and dementia: a quantitative study. Acta Neuropathol. **37** (1977) 111−118.

[3] De Kloet, E. R.: Brain corticosteroid receptor balance and homeostatic control. Front. Neuroendocrinol. **12** (1991) 95−165.

[4] Ferrier, I. N., J. Pascual, B. G. Charlton et al.: Cortisol, ACTH, and dexamethasone concentrations in a psychogeriatric population. Biol. Psychiatry **3** (1988) 252−260.

[5] Halbreich, U., G. M. Asnis, B. Zumoff et al.: Effects of age and sex on cortisol secretion in depressives and normals. Psychiatry Res. **13** (1984) 221−229.

[6] Heuser, I. J., U. Gotthardt, U. Schweiger, J. Schmider, C.-H. Lammers, M. Dettling, F. Holsboer: Age-associated changes of pituitary-adrenocortical hormone regulation in humans: importance of gender. Neurobiol. Aging **15** (1994) 227−231.

[7] Heuser, I. J., U. Gotthardt, U. Schweiger, J. Schmider, C.-H. Lammers, M. Dettling, A. Grasser, F. Holsboer: Pituitary-adrenal-axis regulation and psychopathology during amitriptyline treatment in elderly depressed patients and in normal controls. AmJPsychiatry (subm.).

[8] Heuser, I. J., H.-J. Wark, J. Keul et al.: Hypothalamic-pituitary-adrenal axis function in elderly endurance athletes. J. Clin. Endocrinol. Metab. **73** (1991) 485−488.

[9] Holsboer, F.: Psychiatric implications of altered limbic-hypothalamic-pituitary-adrenocortical activity. Eur. Arch. Psychiatry Neurol. Sci. **238** (1989) 302−322.

[10] Holsboer, F.: Depression. In: R. D. Hesch (ed.) Endokrinologie. Teil B Krankheitsbilder, pp. 1233−1242. Urban & Schwarzenberg, München−Wien−Baltimore 1989.

[11] Holsboer, F., D. Spengler, I. Heuser: The role of corticotropin-releasing hormone in the pathogenesis of Cushing's disease, anorexia nervosa, alcoholism, affective disorders and dementia. In: D. F. Swaab, M. A. Hofman, M. Mirmiran et al. (eds.) Progess in brain research, Vol. 93, pp. 385−417. Elsevier Science Publishers, Amsterdam 1992.

[12] Holsboer-Trachsler, E., R. Stohler, M. Hatzinger: Repeated administration of the combined dexamethasone/hCRH stimulation test during treatment of depression. Psychiatry Res. 38 (1991) 163–171.

[13] Lorens, S. A., N. Hata, R. J. Handa et al.: Neurochemical, endocrine and immunological responses to stress in young and old Fischer 344 male rats. Neurobiol. Aging 11 (1990) 139–150.

[14] Ohashi, M., N. Fujio, H. Nawata et al.: Aging is without effect on the pituitary-adrenal axis in men. Gerontology 32 (1986) 335–339.

[15] Oxenkrug, G. F., N. Pomara, I. M. McIntyre et al.: Aging and cortisol resistance to suppression by dexamethasone: A positive correlation. Psychiatry Res. 10 (1983) 125–130.

[16] Reul, J. M. H. M., J. Tonnaer, R. de Kloet: Neurotrophic ACTH analogue promotes plasticity of Type I corticosteroid receptor in brain of senescent male rats. Neurobiol. Aging 9 (1988) 253–260.

[17] Rolandi, E., R. Franceschini, A. Marabini et al.: Twenty-four-hour beta-endorphin secretory pattern in the elderly. Acta Endocrinol. (Copenh.) 115 (1987) 441–446.

[18] Sapolsky, R. M., J. Altmann: Incidence of hypercortisolism and dexamethasone resistance increases with age among wild baboons. Biol. Psychiatry 30 (1991) 1008–1016.

[19] Sapolsky, R. M., L. C. Krey, B. S. McEwen: The adrenocortical stress-response in the aged male rat: impairment of recovery from stress. Exp. Gerontol. 18 (1983) 55–64.

[20] Sapolsky, R. M., L. C. Krey, B. S. McEwen: Prolonged glucocorticoid exposure reduces hippocampal neuron number: implications for aging. J. Neurosci. 5 (1985) 1222–1227.

[21] Scaccianoce, S., A. di Sciullo, L. Angelucci: Age-related changes in hypothalamo-pituitary-adrenocortical axis activity in the rat. In vitro studies. Neuroendocrinology 52 (1990) 150–155.

[22] Sharma, M., J. Palacios-Bois, G. Schwartz et al.: Circadian rhythms of melatonin and cortisol in aging. Biol. Psychiatry 25 (1989) 305–319.

[23] Van Eekelen, J. A. M., N. Y. Rots, W. Sutanto et al.: The effect of aging on stress responsiveness and central corticosteroid receptors in the Brown Norway rat. Neurobiol. Aging 13 (1991) 159–170.

[24] Von Bardeleben, U., F. Holsboer: Cortisol response to a combined dexamethasone-h-CRH challenge in patients with depression. J. Neuroendocrinol. 1 (1989) 485–488.

[25] Von Bardeleben, U., G. K. Stalla, O. A. Müller et al.: Blunting of ACTH response to human CRH in depressed patients is avoided by metyrapone pretreament. Biol. Psychiatry 24 (1988) 782–786.

[26] Verkhratsky, N. S., E. V. Moroz, L. V. Magdich et al.: Steroid-hormone-secretion-regulating system under effect of stress in old age. Gerontology 34 (1988) 41–47.

[27] Waltman, C., M. R. Blackman, G. P. Chrousos: Spontaneous and glucocorticoid-inhibited adrenocorticotropic hormone and cortisol secretion are similar in healthy young and old men. J. Clin. Endocrinol. Metab. 73 (1991) 495–502.

[28] Zimmerman, M., W. Coryell: The dexamethasone suppression test in healthy controls. Psychoneuroendocrinology 12 (1987) 245–251.

Age-dependent changes in brain neurotransmitters and their influence on neuroendocrine functions

J. Meites

Introduction

From a physiological point of view, aging may be defined as a progressive decline with time in the morphological and functional integrity of organs, tissues, and cells in the body, associated with a decrease in ability to maintain homeostasis. Although it is commonly held that aging begins only in the later years of life, the decline in body functions actually begins much earlier. The pioneer investigations of the late Nathan Shock [27] demonstrated that in humans from the ages of 30 to 90 years there is a progressive decrease in cardiovascular function, pulmonary vital capacity, renal function, nerve conduction velocity, maximum work rate, etc. Similar relatively early declines in body functions occur in animals.

What is responsible for these age related declines in body functions? Many theories have been developed in an attempt to explain why aging occurs, and it is doubtful that any one theory can provide the entire answer. Almost all investigators agree that the genome determines the length of the lifespan in different species, and to some extent within the same species. The length of lifespan and rate of aging are related, but the nature of this relationship is not clear. Environmental factors are also important in aging processes. The genome and environment are believed to operate to a large degree via the neuroendocrine system which regulate (or influence) body functions throughout life. With time faults develop in neuroendocrine mechanisms that are mainly responsible for the decline in many body functions, including decreases in reproduction, protein synthesis, increases in diseases and tumors, decline in immune competence, and other body changes [16, 17].

The neuroendocrine system consists of the hypothalamic portion of the brain, the portal vessels that originate in the median eminence and carry hypophysiotropic hormones from the hypothalamus to the pituitary, and the pituitary and its target glands (thyroid, adrenals, gonads, pancreas, gastrointestinal tract, and thymus and other immune tissues). The hypothalamus contains two agents that are particularly important for controlling pituitary hormone secretion, namely the hypophysiotropic hormones that are released into the portal vessels to act directly on the pituitary, and neurotransmitters that modulate release of the hypophysiotropic into the portal vessels. Hormones secreted by the pituitary and its target glands, as well as environmental stimuli acting via the CNS, can feed back on the hypothalamic neurotransmitter neurons to alter their secretory activity. Although neurotransmitters have many functions in the brain and elsewhere in the body, only their role in aging processes will be considered here.

Sources of brain neurotransmitters and their effects on hormone secretion

The principal neurotransmitters that influence secretion of hypothalamic and pituitary hormones are believed to be two catecholamines (CAs), dopamine (DA) and norepenephrine (NE), serotonin (5-HT), acetylcholine (Ach), and the brain opiates. Many other neurotransmitters also can influence neuroendocrine function, but little is known of their role during aging as compared to the CAs.

The neural cell bodies that secrete DA, NE, and 5-HT are located mainly in the lower brain stem and mescencephalon. Their axons ascend via the medial forebrain bundle to the hypothalamus, striatum, amygdala, hippocampus, and cortex. Terminals of these neurons in the hypothalamus end directly on the neurons that secrete the peptide hormones (GnRH, TRH, GHRH, CRH) that are released from the median eminence into the portal vessels to regulate pituitary hormone secretion. The DA that inhibits prolactin secretion comes mainly from neurons in the arcuate nucleus of the hypothalamus and is released into the portal vessels to act directly on the pituitary. NE in the hypothalamus originates mainly from neurons located in the locus coeruleus and lateral reticular nucleus of the medulla. The neural fibers that carry 5-HT to the hypothalamus come from the raphe nuclei of the lower pons and upper brainstem, and are distributed to the suprachiasmatic nucleus (SCN) and upper brainstem. The SCN and 5-HT are important in regulating circadian and other rhythms, including rhythms in hormone secretion. Brain opiates originate in many areas of the CNS, including the hypothalamus and pituitary. Ach comes from outside the hypothalamus.

The CAs synthesized in the brain and adrenal medulla are formed from the amino acid, tyrosine, by enzymatic steps: tyrosine to L-dopa to DA to NE to epinephrine. Very little epinephrine is present in the brain, including the hypothalamus, as compared to DA and NE, and its role in neuroendocrine function is of minor importance. The rate limiting enzyme in the synthesis of the CAs is tyrosine hydroxylase. Receptors for DA and NE are present on the neurons that secrete the hypophysiotropic hormones and thereby influence their secretion. The CAs are catabolized mainly by Monoamine oxidase (MAO), and to a lesser extent by catechol-O-methyltransferase (COMT). 5-HT is synthesized from the amino acid, tryptophan, via the action of tryptophan hydroxylase. It is catabolized by MAO to form 5-hydroxyindoleacetic acid (5-HIAA). Ach is synthesized from choline and acetyl CoA by the enzyme choline acetyltransferase (CAT), and is catabolized by acetylcholinesterase. The brain opiates are formed from larger precursors and catabolized by specific enzymes.

In the rat, hypothalamic NE has been demonstrated to be the major neurotransmitter that promotes release of GnRH, GHRH, and TRH from the hypothalamus, and these in turn stimulate pituitary secretion of gonadotropins, GH, and TSH [14, 19]. Administration of L-dopa, the precursor of DA, can duplicate the actions of DA whereas the NE agonist, clonidine, can duplicate the effects of NE on secretion of hormones. CA antagonists, such as the neuroleptic drugs, can increase secretion of prolactin, but decrease secretion of gonadotropins and GH. Administration of dopaminergic drugs such as some ergot derivatives, can inhibit prolactin secretion. 5-HT and its agonists promote secretion of prolactin, GH, and ACTH, whereas 5-HT antagonists reduce release of these hormones in response to various stimuli. Ach and its agonists stimulate GH and ACTH secretion and probably inhibit LH secretion. The brain opiates, mainly B-endorphin, the enkephalins, and dynorphin, stimulate GH and prolactin secretion, and inhibit secretion of FSH, LH, and ACTH.

Changes in hypothalamic neurotransmitters with age

The decline in hypothalamic DA and NE secretion with age is associated with many decreases in body functions in rats. Studies reported by us in 1969 [5] and 1973 [21] suggested the CAs may be deficient in the hypothalamus of old rats. When DA and NE concentrations and turnover (activity) in the hypothalamus of old and young rats were compared we found that both were significantly lower in old than in young rats [29]. These changes with age in rats have been widely confirmed.

Simpkins [28] reported that DA concentrations were lower in the median eminence, medial basal hypothalamus, preoptic area-anterior hypothalamus, and striatum of 25−26 month old than in 3−4 month old female rats. NE concentrations were also lower in the preoptic-anterior and medial basal hypothalamus but not in the median eminence or striatum. McIntosh and Westfall [15] found significant reductions in CA accumulation and release **in vitro** from hypothalamic tissue from Fischer F344 rats 11−14 and 21−26 months old as compared to values in rats 2−4 months old. Gregerson and Selmanoff [8] reported less release of tritium labeled DA from synaptosomes from the median eminence and corpus striatum of old than of young rats. Weiland and Wise [35] observed a decrease in 1-adrenergic receptors in the SCN and median eminence by middle age, and in all hypothalamic areas by old age in rats.

Several investigators have reported a decline in CAs in the hypothalamus and other areas of the brain in aging humans. Hornykiewicz [10] found that NE was decreased significantly in the hypothalamus, hippocampus and other regions of the human brain, which he believes may be due to loss of noradrenergic neurons in the locus coeruleus. By the 9th decade, about 25% of the original cell complement is lost in this brain region. Robinson et al. [23] reported a decrease in DA in both the hypothalamus and thalamus of elderly individuals. There is also a significant loss of DA neurons in the nigra striatal region of the brain in rats and man with age, but this has not been found to influence hypothalamic functions.

No significant changes in 5-HT concentrations have been reported in the hypothalamus of aging rats [28] and the same may be true in elderly men. However, in aging rats the decrease in NE changes the ratio of NE to 5-HT and this may be partly responsible for the loss of the surge of LH release that normally occurs every 4 or 5 days to induce ovulation in cycling rats. There is also some evidence that with age Ach and the brain opiates decline in some areas of the brain, including the hypothalamus, and these may influence hormone secretion.

Why do the hypothalamic catecholamines decline with age?

In the rat a significant loss of neurons has been reported in the arcuate nucleus, medial preoptic area, and ventromedial and lateral hypothalamic nuclei of old rats. There is also a considerable loss of NE neurons in the locus coeruleus which supplies most of the NE to the hypothalamus, as already mentioned. Catabolism of the CAs by MAO results in formation of hydroxyl radicals, hydrogen peroxide, superoxide anions, and highly reactive quinones, which have destructive effects on neurons. There is also evidence for a decrease in tyrosine hydroxylase, resulting in lower synthesis of CAs, and an increase in MAO, leading to greater catabolism of CAs in the hypothalamus and other brain regions. Prolonged exposure to estrogen during the many estrous cycles and the continuous exposure to estrogen during the long constant estrous syndrome in the aging rat, also damages neurons in the hypothalamus. Chronic exposure to estrogen in young rats can similarly damage neurons in the arcuate nucleus and medial basal hypothalamus. Thus many factors are responsible for reducing hypothalamic CA activity with age [see 16, 17].

Effects of aging decline in hypothalamic catecholamines on hormone secretion and body functions

Gonadotropins and reproduction

In old rats, the decrease in hypothalamic NE activity has been shown to be associated with reduced GnRH and gonadotropin secretion, resulting in loss of estrous cycles in females and a decline in testosterone secretion in males [16, 17]. The decrease in NE is also associated with a reduction in GHRH, GH and IGF1 secretion, leading to lower protein synthesis. The reduction in hypothalamic NE is also related to the decline in secretion of TRH, TSH, and thyroid hormones in old rats. There is evidence that the decline in GH and thyroid hormone secretion contribute to the reduction in immune competence with age [17]. The decrease in hypothalamic DA activity is believed to be mainly responsible for the progressive rise in prolactin secretion and for development of numerous mammary and pituitary tumors in aging female rats.

Administration of drugs that elevate hypothalamic CA activity in old rats can delay or reverse most of the above mentioned changes in hormone secretion and related declines in body function [16, 17]. In laboratory rats, estrous cycles become irregular at 7−10 months of age, and cycles usually cease between 10−15 months of age when they enter a constant estrous state characterized by ovarian follicular development but no ovulation. Subsequently, some of the rats exhibit prolonged pseudopregnancies characterized by the presence of numerous corpora lutea in the ovaries. In the final stage of life, between 2−3 years of age, most rats enter into an anestrous state characterized by ovarian atrophy. A remarkable feature of ovaries in these aging rats is that despite a progressive loss of follicles and ova with time, at least some of them remain to the end of life and can be reactivated by gonadotropic hormone stimulation. In aging rats, neither the ovaries nor pituitary are mainly responsible for the declines in reproductive function. It has been demonstrated that when the ovaries of old non-cycling rats are transplanted to young ovarectomized rats, many of the young rats resume cycling [1]. Also, when the pituitary of old rats is transplanted to young hypophysectomized rats, some of the young rats resume cycling [20]. Thus the decline in reproductive functions in rats is due mainly to faults that develop in the hypothalamus. However, the pituitary and gonads become less responsive to hormonal stimulation with age, which contributes to the reproductive decline.

Administration to old rats of L-dopa, the precursor of CAs, or of iproniazid, a MAO inhibitor, was found to induce resumption of estrous cycles in old constant estrous rats [21]. Administration of an ergot drug to reduce the high prolactin secretion in old pseudopregnant rats also resulted in reinitiation of estrous cycles in these animals [4]. Daily feeding of L-dopa to aging rats still exhibiting regular or irregular estrous cycling was shown to delay loss of cycling activity. Lesions placed in the anterior hypothalamus or SCN produce a constant estrous state in mature cycling rats [4], suggesting that this area is essential for maintenance of estrous cycles. Other evidence pointing to the importance of hypothalamic CAs for maintenance of estrous cycles, is that administration of neuroleptic drugs (reserpine, phenathiazines, haloperidol) to young rats reduces brain and hypothalamic CAs, and results in loss of estrous cycles and an increase in prolactin secretion and mammary growth stimulation. Chronic administration of neuroleptic drugs to women has been reported to similarly lead to cessation of menstrual cycles and elevation of prolactin secretion with stimulation of breast growth and even some lactation [14].

Although hypothalamic dysfunction in old rats is mainly responsible for loss of estrous cycles, faults also develop in the pituitary and ovaries (and testes in males). Pituitary release of LH in response to administration of GnRH is lower in old than in young female and male rats [16, 17]. This was found not to be due to loss of GnRH receptors in the pituitary, but to failure of calcium mobilization [25]. There is also evidence that the gonads of old rats become less responsive to the action of gonadotropic hormones. It is clear, however, that these faults are secondary to those that occur in the hypothalamus.

Although there is a decline in hypothalamic CAs in aging humans [10, 23], this does not appear to be a major cause for cessation of menstrual cycles in women or the decrease in testosterone secretion in men. In aging men and women defects that develop in the ovaries and testes are mainly responsible for the reproductive decline [9, 14]. In women approaching the menopause, the ovaries become progressively less responsive to gonadotropic hormone stimulation and show reductions in estrogen secretion, resulting in elevated secretion of FSH and LH. The ovaries atrophy in the postmenopausal period, estrogen secretion is further reduced, and secretion of FSH and LH is further elevated. In men the decreased ability of the testes to secrete testosterone also results in a rise in secretion of gonadotropic hormones. This does not mean that the hypothalamus of elderly individuals is functioning normally [24].

GH secretion and protein synthesis

GH is the most important protein anabolic agent in the body, and is essential for maintaining protein synthesis throughout life. It appears to act mainly by stimulating IGF-1 secretion by the liver and other tissues. The GH decline with age has been confirmed in rats [30, 31], and man [7], and is believed to be at least partly responsible for the decrease in size and function of many body organs and tissues, including the liver, kidneys, GI tract, bone, muscle, skin, and immune tissues.

GH secretion is normally controlled by two hypothalamic hormones, GHRH which increases GH secretion and somatostatin which inhibits GH secretion. There is some evidence that GHRH release is reduced whereas somatostatin release is increased with age [30]. Both DA and especially NE have been demonstrated to promote GH secretion in animals and man, presumably by increasing GHRH release and perhaps also by decreasing somatostatin release. The decrease in hypothalamic CAs with age is believed to be mainly responsible for the decline in GH secretion, as demonstrated by reports showing that administration of L-dopa or clonidine to old rats [30] fully restores GH secretion in these animals. Whether the decline in hypothalamic CAs is responsible to any degree for the decrease in GH secretion in aging humans remains to be determined.

In addition to the decline in hypothalamic stimulation of GH secretion with age, there is also evidence that the pituitary response to GHRH administration in rats and man is reduced [30]. This appears to be due to increased release of somatostatin with age, since under *in vitro* conditions pituitary tissue from old rats releases as much GH in response to GHRH stimulation as pituitary tissue from young rats [30].

Administration of GH or L-dopa was reported to promote protein synthesis in diaphragm muscle in old rats and to significantly increase the weight of the liver, kidneys, heart, thymus and spleen [30]. Elevation of GH levels in old rats was also shown to restore size and function of the thymus, the chief component of the immune system, in old rats [12]. In men 60−80 years of age injections of GH for six months significantly increased lean body mass, reduced adipose tissue mass, increased skin thickness, and produced a small increase in density of lumbar vertebral bone [26].

Prolactin secretion and development of pituitary and mammary tumors

In old female rats and mice the incidence of spontaneous mammary and pituitary tumors is very high. Development of mammary tumors in old Sprague-Dawley females may reach 80% and pituitary tumors are as high as 50%. The occurrence of mammary tumors in female mice of the inbred C3H strain is 80−90%. Prolactin and estrogen are both essential hormones for development of mammary tumors in rats and mice. Pituitary tumors in these species are mainly composed of prolactin cells (prolactinomas). In aging female rats a progressive rise in prolactin secretion occurs mainly due to the decrease in DA inhibition from the hypothalamus, and perhaps also because of high estrogen secretion during the prolonged constant estrous syndrome [16]. Estrogen was shown to stimulate prolactin secretion by acting directly on the pituitary and by damaging DA secreting neurons in the arcuate nucleus.

Administration of drugs such as L-dopa and iproniazid that raise hypothalamic CAs in old rats can induce regression of mammary and pituitary tumors by reducing prolactin secretion [16, 17]. Prolonged administration of bromocryptine to C3H mice was shown to almost completely inhibit development of mammary adenocarcinomas in this high tumor strain [34].

In women prolactin does not appear to have an important role in development of breast tumors. There is actually a slight fall in prolactin secretion in postmenopausal women, presumably due to the decrease in estrogen secretion. Prolactinomas that develop in humans to not appear to be related to changes in hypothalamic DA activity although this requires further investigation [14].

Effects of elevating hypothalamic catecholamines on other body functions in aging animals

The incidence of disease and tumors is known to increase with age. Are these related to the reduction in hypothalamic CAs with age? Walker et al. [32] studied the effects of daily administration of ibopamine, a catecholaminergic drug that stimulates DA and NE receptors, on development of neoplastic and non-neoplastic diseases. The neoplastic diseases studied were tumors of the adrenal cortex, pituitary and mammary glands, skin papillomas, and pheochromocytoma. The non-neoplastic diseases were chronic glomerulonephropathy, renal pelvic mineralization, hepatocellular proliferative nodule, galactoceles, and chronic cardiomyopathy, all common diseases in old rats. Ibopamine treatment was begun at 50 days of age and continued for 2 years. The incidence of all neoplastic and non-neoplastic diseases was significantly reduced in the drug-treated as compared to the control rats. There were no significant differences in food intake or body weight between the ibopamine and control groups, except for a slight decrease in body weight in the rats given the highest does of ibopamine. A reduction in food intake has been demonstrated to decrease the incidence of disease and tumors in rats, mice and other species [33]. The actions of ibopamine cannot be attributed to reduced food intake.

Several investigators have reported that drugs that elevate brain CA levels can prolong the lifespan of rats or mice. Cotzias et al. [6] found that administration of L-dopa in the diet of Swiss albino mice increased their average lifespan by about 50% and extended their period of fertility. However, the mice showed decreased body weight, suggesting that reduced food intake was probably responsible for these results. Clemens and Fuller [4] fed lergotrile mesylate, a DA receptor agonist, for two years to female rats. In two separate experiments, only 40 and 50% of control rats were still alive at the end of two years whereas 70 and 90% of the drug treated rats were still alive at the end of two years. This drug produced no adverse effect on food intake or on body weight.

The most dramatic effects of a catecholaminergic drug on lifespan in rats was reported by Knoll [13]. He injected deprenyl, a MAO-B inhibitor, three times weekly, to 66 two year old males, and injected physiological saline to 66 control male rats. The average lifespan of the deprenyl treated rats was 198 weeks (3.8 years) compared to only 147 weeks (2.8 years) in the control rats. The lifespan of the deprenyl treated rats was stated to exceed the normal maximum lifespan of these animals. In addition, deprenyl was reported to increase the sexual performance of the male rats, suggesting a relation between sexual performance and length of lifespan in male rats. No information on body weight or food intake was provided. These effects of deprenyl of lifespan were partially confirmed in a study by Milgram et al. [18] in two year old male Fischer F344 rats, a shorter-lived inbred strain than the longer-lived hybrid strain used by Knoll [13]. Lifespan in these rats was prolonged only for a few months by deprenyl. Body weight in the deprenyl-treated rats was not significantly different than in the controls, suggesting that the effects on lifespan were not due to reduced food intake. Ephedrine and phenylephrine also were reported to increase survival and reduce occurrence of leukemia and pheochromocytoma in Fischer 344/N rats and B6C3F1 mice [3, 11]. All of these reports on the effects of catecholaminergic drugs are of great interest and may have important implications for aging humans. However, further studies are necessary to confirm the results reported and to further clarify the mode(s) of action of these drugs.

Conclusions

It is clear that the decrease in the two CAs, DA and NE, in the hypothalamus of aging rats is associated with a decline in release of a number of hypothalamic hypophysiotropic hormones, resulting in reduced secretion by the pituitary of gonadotropins, GH, TSH, and increased secretion of prolactin. These result in reduced reproductive functions, decreased protein synthesis, lower thyroid hormone secretion and reduced body metabolism, occurrence of numerous mammary and pituitary tumors, and decreased immune competence. It is probable that the decreases in GH and thyroid hormone secretion contribute to many other declines in body function with age.

If the decrease in hypothalamic CAs in rats contributes importantly to the aging decline in body functions, can a reduction in hypothalamic CAs in young or mature rats reproduce or hasten these declines in body functions? The answer appears to be at least partially in the affirmative. Administration of neuroleptic drugs (reserpine, penothiazines, haloperidol, etc.) that decrease brain CAs to young or mature rats (and other species) results in decreased gonadotropin secretion and cessation of estrous cycles, reduced secretion of GH, and increased secretion of prolactin and early development of mammary tumors. Other decreases in body functions may be produced by chronic administration of drugs that decrease hypothalamic CAs. These results in young or mature rats further emphasize the importance of hypothalamic CAs in aging processes, and suggest that changes in hypothalamic functions per se rather than age may be the determining factors in many declines in body functions.

Administration of catecholaminergic drugs to old rats can delay or reverse many of the declines in body functions normally observed in aging rats. Such drugs were observed to reinitiate estrous cycles, elevate GH secretion and promote protein synthesis, induce regression of mammary and pituitary tumors, inhibit incidence of other diseases, increase male sexual behavior, and even prolong the lifespan. Other neurotransmitters in the hypothalamus may also have a role in aging developments, although there is little information on these at present. Other changes inside and outside of the hypothalamus, including reduced responsiveness of the pituitary and its target glands to hormonal stimuli, may also contribute to the aging process. In general, the studies reported here appear to confirm the view that heredity and environment regulate aging processes largely via the neuroendocrine system.

The role of hypothalamic CAs on hormone secretion and body functions in elderly humans is largely unknown. CAs are lower in old than in young individuals [10, 11], probably due to the significant loss of NE neurons in the locus coeruleus. There is loss of DA neurons in the arcuate nucleus. The reduction of dopaminergic neurons in the substantia nigra and of cholinergic neurons in the hippocampus do not appear to directly influence hypothalamic hormone secretion. The decline in hypothalamic CAs in aging individuals may be responsible for the decrease in GH secretion, although this remains to be demonstrated. Both L-dopa and clonidine, a NE agonist, have been shown to elevate GH secretion in man [14]. Deprenyl given together with L-dopa and a peripheral inhibitor of L-dopa metabolism was reported to prolong the lifespan of patients with Parkinson's disease [2].

A preliminary study on the effects of administering deprenyl for 12 weeks to rats indicated that it significantly increased NE and 5-HT concentrations in the hypothalamus, but had no effect on DA concentration (Quadri, unpublished data). Serum prolactin levels were reduced in these deprenyl-treated rats, as was reported in an early study when rats were injected with iproniazid, another MAO inhibitor [21]. Whether catecholaminergic drugs will prove to be useful for delaying or reversing aging processes in humans remains to be investigated. Since there is evidence that with age other neurotransmitters are reduced in some regions of the brain, including acetylcholine, it would be of interest to determine the effects on body functions in old rats given a combination of drugs that increase brain neurotransmitters.

References

[1] Aschheim, P.: Relation of the neuroendocrine system to reproductive declines in female rats. In: J. Meites (ed.) Neurobiology of aging, pp. 73–101. Plenum Press, New York 1983.

[2] Birkmeyer, W., J. G. D. Birkmeyer: The L-dopa story. In: D. B. Caine, C. G. Crippa, R. Horowski, et al. [eds.] Parkinsonism and Aging, pp. 1–7. Raven Press, New York 1989.

[3] Buckner, J. R.: Toxicology and carcinogenesis studies of ephenephrine hydrochloride in F344/N rats and B6C3F1 mice. Technical Report Series no. 307, National Toxicology Program, Research Triangle Park, North Carolina, 1986.

[4] Clemens, J. A., Fuller, R. W.: Chemical manipulation of some aspects of aging. In: R. Roberts, R. C. Adelman, V. J. Cristofalo (eds.) Pharmacological interventions in the aging process, pp. 187–206. Plenum Press, New York 1977.

[5] Clemens, J. A., Y. Amenomori, T. Jenkins et al.: Effects of hypothalamic stimulation, hormones, and drugs on ovarian function in old female rats. Proc. Soc. Exp. Biol. and Med. 132 (1969) 561–563.

[6] Cotzias, G., S. Miller, A. Nicholson Jr. et al.: Levodopa, fertility, and longevity. Proc. Nat. Acad. Sci. USA 71 (1974) 2466–2469.

[7] Florini, J. R., P. N. Prinz, M. V. Vitiello et al.: Somatomedin-C levels in healthy young and old men: Relationships to peak and 24-hour integrated levels of growth hormone. J. Gerontology 40 (1985) 2–7.

[8] Gregerson, K. A., Selmanoff, M.: Changes in the kinetics of ^{3}H dopamine release from median eminence and striatal synaptosomes during aging. Endocrinology 126 (1990) 228–234.

[9] Harman, S. M.: Clinical aspects of the male reproductive system. In: E. L. Schneider (ed.) The aging reproductive system, pp. 29–58. Raven Press, New York 1978.

[10] Hornykiewicz, O.: Neurotransmitter changes in the human brain. In: S. Govoni, F. Battaini (eds.) Modification of cell to cell signals during normal and pathological aging, pp. 169–182. Springer Verlag, Berlin–Heidelberg 1987.

[11] Irwin, R.: Toxicology and carcinogenesis studies of ephedrine sulfate in F344/N rats and B6C3F1 mice. Technical Report Series no. 307, National Toxicology Program, Research Triangle Park, North Carolina 1986.

[12] Kelly, K. W., S. Brief, H. J: Westley et al.: GH3 pituitary adenoma cells can reverse thymic aging in rats. Proc. Nat. Acad. Sci. USA 83 (1986) 5666–5667.

[13] Knoll, J.: The striatal dopamine dependency of lifespan in male rats. Longevity study with (-)deprenyl. Mechanisms of Aging and Development 46 (1988) 237–262.

[14] Martin, J. B., S. Reichlin: Clinical Neuroendocrinology, 2nd edition. F. A. Davis, Philadelphia 1987.

[15] McIntosh, J.: Regional changes in monoamine metabolism in the aging constant estrous rat. Neurobiology of Aging 4 (1982) 3309–3314.

[16] Meites, J.: Neuroendocrine basis of aging in the rat. In: A. A. Everitt, J. R. Walton (eds.) Regulation of neuroendocrine aging, pp. 37–50. Karger, Basel 1988.

[17] Meites, J.: Aging: hypothalamic catecholamines, neuroendocrine-immune interactions, and dietary restriction. Proc. Soc. Exp. Biol. & Med. 195 (1990) 304–311.

[18] Milgram, N. W., R. J. Racine, P. Nellis et al.: Maintenance on L-deprenyl prolongs life in aged male rats. Life Sciences 47 (1990) 415–420.

[19] Müller, E. E., G. Nistico, U. Scapagnini: Neurotransmitter and anterior pituitary function. Academic Press, Inc., New York 1977.

[20] Peng, M. T.: Changes in hormone uptake and receptors in the hypothalamus during aging. In: J. Meites (ed.) Neurobiology of Aging, pp. 61–72. Plenum Press, New York 1983.

[21] Quadri, S. K., G. S. Kledzik, J. Meites: Reinitiation of estrous cycles in old constant estrous rats by central acting drugs. Neuroendocrinology 11 (1973) 248–255.

[22] Quadri, S. K., D. Palazzolo: How aging affects the canine endocrine system. Veterinary Medicine (July, 1991) 692–702.

[23] Robinson, D. S., A. Nies, J. Davis et al.: Aging, monoamines and monoamine oxidase levels. Lancet i (1972) 290–291.

[24] Rossmanith, W. F., W. A. Scherbaum, C. Lauritzen: Gonadotropin secretion during aging in post menopausal women. Neuroendocrinology 54 (1991) 211–218.

[25] Roth, G. S.: Changes in hormone action with age: altered calcium mobilization and/or responsiveness impairs signal transduction. In: H. J. Armbrecht, R. M. Coe, N. Wongsurawal (eds.) Endocrine function and aging, pp. 26–34. Springer Verlag, New York 1990.

[26] Rudman, D., A. G. Feller, S. N. Hoskote et al.: Effects of human growth hormone in men over 60 years old. New England J. of Med. 323 (1990) 1–6.

[27] Shock, N.: System integration. In: C. F. Finch, L. Hayflick (eds.) Handbook of the biology of aging, pp. 639–665. Van Nostrand Reinhold, New York, 1977.

[28] Simpkins, J. W.: Changes in hypothalamic hypophysiotropic hormones and neurotransmitters during aging. In: J. Meites (ed.) Neuroendocrinology of aging, pp. 41–59. Plenum Press, New York, 1983.

[29] Simpkins, J. W., G. P. Mueller, H. H. Huang et al.: Evidence for depressed catecholamine and enhanced serotonin metabolism in aging male rats; possible relation to gonadotropin secretion. Endocrinology 100 (1977) 1672–1678.

[30] Sonntag, W. E., Meites, J.: Decline in growth hormone secretion in aging animales and man. In: A. V. Everitt, J. R. Walton (eds.) Regulation of neuroendocrine aging, pp. 111–124. Karger, Basel 1988.

[31] Sonntag, W. E., R. W. Steger, L. J. Forman et al.: Decreased pulsatile release of growth hormone in old male rats. Endocrinology 107 (1980) 1875–1879.

[32] Walker, R. F., C. A. Weideman, E. B. Wheeldon et al.: Reduced disease in aged rats treated chronically with ibopamine, a catecholaminergic drug. Neurobiology of Aging 9 (1988) 291–301.

[33] Weindruch, R. R., I. Walford: The retardation of aging and disease by dietary restriction. Charles C. Thomas, Springfield, Il. 1988.

[34] Welsch, C. W., H. Nagasawa: Prolactin and murine tumorigenesis. A review. Cancer Research 37 (1977) 951–963.

[35] Weiland, N. G., Wise, P. M.: Aging progressively decreases the densities and alters the diurnal rhythm of 1-adrenergic receptors in selected hypothalamic regions. Endocrinology 126 (1990) 2392–2397.

Thirst and osmoregulation in the elderly

J. Hensen

Introduction

The normal aging process is accompanied by changes in water content of the body. Total body water decreases due primarily to an increase in body fat but also to a decline in hydration of lean body mass [41]. These water losses affect both intracellular and extracellular compartments. The decrease in total body water in people who have "aged sucessfully" does not necessarily lead to an increase in extracellular tonicity [28] as long as the osmoregulatory system is intact. However, the function of the osmoregulatory system and thus, also, the tonicity regulation of the extracellular fluid are likewise subject to changes with age. Before these changes are outlined, the mechanisms of the osmoregulatory system will be briefly recapitulated.

Blood tonicity is osmolality corrected for the relative cell permeability of the individual solutes. Osmolality and tonicity are identical for sodium, the major solute of the blood, but not for urea and glucose [9, 46]. The body regulates blood tonicity by adding water to or extracting it from the blood and excreting it via the kidneys (like a cook thickening a sauce by boiling it down or thinning it by adding water). The **antidiuretic hormone (ADH)**, i. e. arginine-vasopressin (AVP), is in charge of regulating water output from the kidneys.

An increasing extracellular tonicity, primarily caused by an increase in plasma sodium, is sensed by the osmoreceptor neurons. The osmoreceptors seem to be located at the anteroventral portion of the third cerebral ventricle, probably in the organum vasculosum laminae terminalis (OVLT). The osmoreceptor neurons transmit information to the cerebral cortex by poorly defined pathways, thus triggering the perception of **thirst**. The desire for water is communicated or another water-seeking behavior is induced. A certain amount of water is drunk, overload being prevented by pharyngeal and gastric reflexes [1, 4]. Finally, water is absorbed from the gut.

The osmoreceptor neurons also send their signals to the magnocellular neurons of the supraoptic and paraventricular nuclei to release **ADH** from the posterior pituitary. Vasopressin (VP) secretion is usually closely dependent on plasma tonicity, the threshold osmolality being about $285-290$ mosmol/kg (Fig. 1). ADH reaches the kidney via the bloodstream. Vasopressin V_2-receptors are located on the principal cells of the collecting ducts. The binding of ADH to these

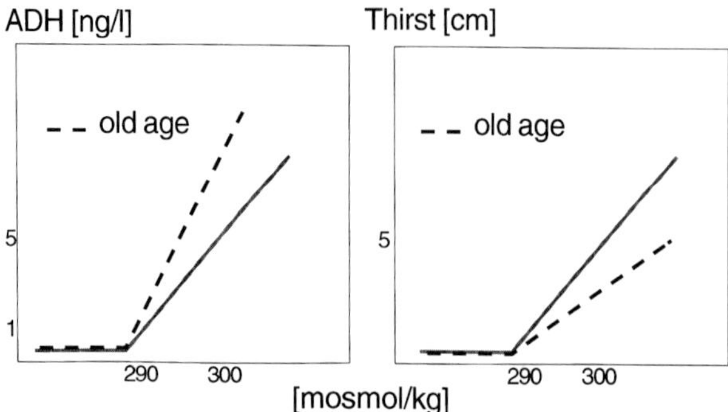

Fig. 1   Dependence of plasma ADH and thirst on plasma osmolality.

receptors stimulates cAMP generation, which subsequently activates protein kinases and thereby increases the hydraulic conductivity of the cells. The interstitial medullary osmolality in the kidney is usually above 1000 mosmol/kg due to the countercurrent mechanism. The presence of VP thus permits water to cross the tubular cells from the luminal to the intramedullary site along the osmotic gradient. Finally, vasopressin is degraded in, for example, the liver and kidney.

A variety of hormones act in concert to modulate these different processes. Angiotensin II seems to increase thirst, at least in rats, but some evidence has also pointed to a role in humans with severe renal-artery stenosis. The atrial natriuretic factor (ANF) inhibits not only the release [3] but also the action of vasopressin [7]. In addition, vasopressin release is subject to tonic inhibition by cortisol [11].

The pathways delineated above can be interrupted or disturbed at any stage. For example, destruction of the osmoreceptor by bleeding into an aneurysm of the anterior communicating artery might abolish ADH secretion and thirst, thus leading to severe hypernatremia [cf. 18]. Increased degradation of vasopressin, as in pregnancy, might uncover previously compensated diabetes insipidus [cf. 19]. Hypovolemia increases vasopressin secretion via baroreceptor activation and presumably also via a plasma ANF decrease.

Disturbances of vasopressin **action** might also occur anywhere in the system: in the VP binding, in the intracellular signalling mechanism, in the formation and action of aquaphores and also in the intramedullary osmotic gradient.

Alterations of thirst with aging

Thirst sensation in the elderly is reduced to certain stimuli, such as water deprivation [36], heat stress [29], or hypertonic saline infusion [35]. Reduced thirst is detectable even in the absence of preexisting cerebrovascular disease. Why the elderly show reduced thirst sensitivity is unclear. Thirst sensation was reported to be diminished by activation of high- and low-pressure baroreceptors and by the atrial natriuretic hormone (ANH). However, baroreceptor sensitivity is also reduced with age, and plasma levels of cGMP, the second messenger of ANP, are not necessarily elevated in the elderly [34]. Some authors have suggested impaired angiotensin II production in elderly patients as the cause of their diminished thirst perception [45]. It seems likely that most of the thirst deficit in the elderly is central, possibly originating in the efferent thirst pathways from the osmoreceptor neurons.

Alterations of ADH-secretion with aging

Several studies have shown alterations of ADH concentrations in the brain. In different areas of the brain, including the hypothalamo-hypophyseal system and CSF, VP levels seem to decline during the aging process [cf. 23]. Conflicting results have been reported on the basal ADH plasma levels in the elderly [31]. Several authors [13, 24, 38] have observed a progressive plasma ADH increase with age that becomes most evident in subjects over 60 [13]. Other authors found no plasma ADH differences between young and old subjects [17, 40]. All studies demonstrated, however, that an osmotic challenge (intravenous hypertonic saline infusion) in the elderly resulted in a greater increase of plasma ADH in response to the rise in serum osmolality than in younger subjects [17]. Also, after intravenous ethanol, the decline in plasma ADH was less marked in the older than in the younger subjects [17]. The observations were interpreted as indicating greater osmoreceptor sensitivity as a consequence of aging. It was suggested that the impaired baroreceptor input to the supraoptic nucleus in the elderly [40] may be the basis for the enhanced ADH response to an osmotic stimulus [16].

There is also some evidence that an increased activity of endogenous opioids in the elderly might mediate increased synthesis and release of ADH [12]. Indeed, administration of the nonselective opioid receptor antagonist naloxone has been shown to normalize both water excretion and diluting capacity in elderly patients [31].

Alterations of renal concentrating capacity with aging

The mechanism of water conservation is impaired in the aging human. It has been demonstrated by numerous authors that maximal urine concentration is

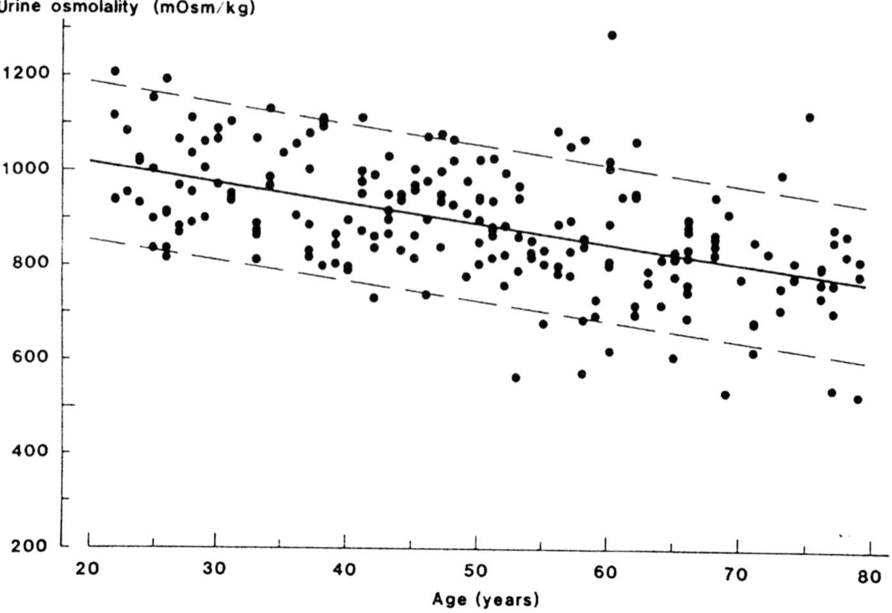

Fig. 2   Pak urine osmolality after DDAVP as a function of age in 211 healthy adults. Fluid was withheld from 10:00 p. m. the night before, and 150 ml fluid was allowed in the morning. At 8:00 a. m., the bladder was emptied, and DDAVP was administered as a 4 µg s. c. injection in the upper arm. No fluid was allowed between 8:00 a. m. and 11:00 a. m. Urine was collected 1 h, 3 h and 6 h after DDAVP administration. From [44].

impaired in the elderly [26]. In a recent study by Tryding and colleagues (Fig. 2), peak urine osmolality after DDAVP ranged from 982 ± 214 mosmol/kg (mean ± 2 SD) at 20 years to 823 ± 278 mosmol/kg at 80 years [44].

Why is the effect of ADH on the kidney impaired in the elderly [30]? Possible explanations for the decreased renal concentrating capacity include a washout of medullary tonicity due to a relative increase in renal medullary blood flow [27]. Also, an increase in solute load per nephron due to nephron dropout with advanced age will result in an obligate osmotic diuresis [30, 43]. Moreover, a decline in glomerular filtration rate (GFR) [25, 44] and an increased incidence of renal disease with advanced age might contribute to the impaired ability to conserve water [43]. Finally, it was discussed that the impaired renal concentrating capacity might be partly due to the high prevalence of bacteriuria in elderly patients [8, 43].

Examinations of renal V_2-vasopressin **receptors** have yielded conflicting results. On the one hand, primary renal-cell preparations from young and old mice were found to have identical receptor concentrations [5]. On the other hand, a decrease in renal binding sites has been demonstrated for ADH in aged rats by a membrane-binding assay [21] and an immunocytochemical staining procedure [37]. Herzberg et al. [21] reported that testosterone treatment could restore these reduced vasopressin-binding sites. However, testosterone treatment failed to improve the renal concentrating capacity [15], suggesting that postreceptor events might also be impaired with aging [5]. This was confirmed by experiments in mice and rats. The cAMP response of rat renal papillary slices to ADH was decreased [2]. Moreover, a higher threshold dose of ADH was required to elicit a significant cAMP rise in old animals, and the dose response curve was shifted to the right in old mice [14]. As receptor affinity and density were unchanged, it was concluded that the decreased cAMP response is probably associated with post-receptor mechanisms [5]. However, more work is needed using newer vasopressin ligands with high specific radioactivity [10] and molecular techniques to clarify this situation.

What is the connection between enhanced osmoreceptor sensitivity (and thus also ADH secretion) and renal ADH resistance? It has been proposed that the decrease in renal ADH receptors with its resultant impaired renal concentrating capacity and water loss might be the cause of the hypothalamo-neurohypophyseal activation in senescence [31]. According to this proposal, the increased AVP secretion reflects the decreased collecting-tubule sensitivity to AVP. The sensitivity changes is not completely offset by increased ADH release, and this reduces the concentrating capacity [6]. Conversely, increased ADH secretion could be the primary event resulting from aging affects on the hypothalamus and central nervous system. Miller [31] demonstrated that chronic exposure to moderately elevated vasopressin levels impaired kidney responsiveness to its antidiuretic action both in vivo and in vitro, perhaps through downregulation of V_2-vasopressin receptors. They concluded that the increase in ADH secretion that occurs with age is responsible for the altered renal ADH responsiveness. This was supported by data on heterozygote Brattleboro rats that have only half the ADH secretory capacity of normal rats. These rats display maintenance of concentrating capacity throughout life [31].

Alterations of renal diluting capacity with aging

Free water clearance has been shown to be intact in older subjects with a preserved GFR [6]. Those with an age-related decresae in GFR usually still dilute their urine sufficiently (< 100 mosm/kg) to ensure solute-free water intake without occurrence of plasma hypo-osmolality [6].

Effect of aging on other hormones involved in osmoregulation

Water economy is also altered by a variety of hormones besides vasopressin. Most of these hormones are volume regulators and thus only play a secondary

Table 1   Effect of aging on hormones involved in water balance (adapted from [32]).

Hormone	Age-related change in serum level	Possible age-related effect on electrolytes
ADH-basal	increased	Hyponatremia
ADH-osmotic stimulated	increased	Hyponatremia
ADH-Baroreceptor stimulated	decreased	Hypernatremia
Atrial natriuretic hormone	increased	Hyponatremia
PRA/Angiotensin II/Aldosterone	decreased	Hyponatremia, hypernatremia (decrease of thirst?), hyperkalemia
ACTH-basal	normal	no effect
Cortisol-basal	normal	no effect
Thyroid hormones-basal	normal	no effect

role in osmoregulation (Tab. 1). ANH is a natriuretic and vasodilative hormone secreted by the heart in response to an atrial dilation. It is also stimulated by AVP. Plasma concentrations of ANH are slightly increased in aged men [34], but not necessarily the concentration of its second messenger cGMP. Plasma renin activity and plasma aldosterone are also reduced with age, thus predisposing elderly to hyperkalemia.

Clinical implications

Manifest dysnatremias are normally not seen in "well-off older people". The most frequent osmoregulatory disturbance in the impaired elderly is **hypernatremia** [20, 39, 43, 45]. The condition is well known in dehydrated nursing home patients; its presence indicates clinical neglect [22]. Snyder et al. [43] examined hypernatremia in an elderly population and found the most frequent primary causes to the incomplete replacement of water loss due to surgical complications, febrile illness, infirmity and diabetes mellitus. Notably, sensorium depression correlated with the severity of hypernatremia. Hyperosmolality is a marker for increased mortality [33]. The frequency of **hyponatremia** is also increased in the elderly. Sodium and water losses such as those caused by diarrhea or **diuretic therapy**, can result in **hypovolemia** and diminish fluid delivery to the distal diluting segments of the nephron. Hypovolemia also stimulates vasopressin, and water is retained even at the expense of hypoosmolality. A decreased effective arterial blood pressure, as in congestive heart failure, liver cirrhosis, and nephrotic syndrome, will also lead to dilutional hyponatremia. In addition, hyponatremia might result from the limited excretion of a solute-free water load in advanced chronic renal failure [42]. Rarely, an inappropiate secretion of ADH (SIADH), e. g. by a bronchogenic carcinoma, might cause hyponatremia.

Conclusion

Reduced thirst as well as an **impairment of renal concentration capacity** in the elderly might predispose them to significant dehydration and **hypernatremia,** especially under conditions of limited water access (physical incapacity, illness, drug sedation) or increased water loss (fever, hot weather) [20, 43]. It may be that obligatory fluid intake may be helpful in preventing dehydration and reducing morbidity under such conditions [35]. It is not yet completely understood whether the exaggerated release of ADH in response to an osmotic challenge favors the development of hyponatremia in certain conditions, such as congestive heart failure. This is unlikely, however, since ADH release by the baroreceptor mechanism has been shown to be decreased in the elderly. Intake of drugs that reduce free water clearance (e. g. diuretics) and volume depletion are the two primary causes of hyponatremia in the elderly [6].

References

[1]   Appelgren, B. H., T. N. Thrasher, L. C. Keil et al.: Mechanism of drinking-induced inhibition of vasopressin secretion in dehydrated dogs. Am. J. Physiol. Regul. Integr. Comp. Physiol. **261** (1991) R1226−R1233.

[2]   Beck, N., B. P. Yu: Effect of aging on urinary concentrating mechanism and vasopressin-dependent cAMP in rats. Am. J. Physiol. **243** (1982) 121−125.

[3]   Clark, B. A., D. Elahi, L. Fish et al.: Atrial natriuretic peptide suppresses osmostimulated vasopressin release in young and elderly humans. Am. J. Physiol. Endocrinol. Metab. **261** (1991) E252−E256.

[4]   Cowart, B. J.: Development of taste perception in humans: sensitivity and preference throughout the lifespan. Psychol. Bull. **90** (1981) 43−73.

[5]   Davidson, Y. S., I. Davies, C. Goddard: Renal vasopressin receptors in aging C57BL/Icrfa[†] mice. J. Endocrinol. **115** (1987) 379−385.

[6]   Davis, P. J., F. B. Davis: Water excretion in the elderly. Endocrinol. Metabol. Clin. North Am. **16** (1987) 867−875.

[7]   Dillingham, M. A., R. J. Anderson: Inhibition of vasopressin action by atrial natriuretic factor. Science **231** (1986) 1572−1573.

[8]   Dontas, A. S., P. Papanayiotou, S. G. Marketos et al.: The effect of bacteriuria on renal functional patterns in old age. Clin. Sci. **34** (1968) 73−81.

[9]   Dürr, J., W. H. Hoffman, J. Hensen et al.: Osmoregulation of vasopressin in diabetic ketoacidosis. Am. J. Physiol. **259** (1990) E723−E728.

[10] Dürr, J. A., J. Hensen, R. W. Schrier: High specific activity ^{125}I- and ^{35}S-labeled vasopressin analogues with high affinity for the V_1 and V_2 vasopressin isoreceptors. J. Biol. Chem. **267** (1992) 18453−18458.

[11] Escrig, C., A. E. Bishop, H. Inagaki et al.: Localisation of endothelin like immunoreactivity in adult and developing human gut. Gut **33** (1992) 212−217.

[12] Forsling, M.: Opioids in vasopressin release. In: A. W. Jr. Cowley, J. F. Liard, D. A. Ausiello (eds.): Vasopressin − Cellular and integrative functions, pp. 371−377. Raven Press, New York 1989.

[13] Frolkis, V. V., S. F. Golovchenko, V. I. Medved et al.: Vasopressin and cardiovascular system in aging. Gerontology **28** (1982) 290−302.

[14] Goddard, C., Y. S. Davidson, B. B. Moser et al.: Effect of aging on cyclic AMP output by renal medullary cells in response to arginine vasopressin in vitro in C57BL/Icrfa[†] mice. J. Endocrinol. **103** (1984) 133−139.

[15] Goudsmit, E., E. Fliers, D. F. Swaab: Vasopressin and oxytocin excretion in the Brown-Norway rat in relation to aging, water metabolism and testosterone. Mechanisms of Aging and Development **44** (1988) 241−252.

[16] Hamon, G., S. Jouquey: Kappa agonists and vasopressin secretion. Horm. Res. **34** (1990) 129−132.

[17] Helderman, J. H., R. W. Vestal, J. W. Rowe et al.: The response of arginine vasopressin to intravenous ethanol and hypertonic saline in man: The impact of aging. J. Gerontol. **33** (1978) 39−47.

[18] Hensen, J., V. Bähr, W. Oelkers: Schwere Hypernatriämie bei erworbener Störung der Durst- und Vasopressinregulation (Severe hypernatremia due to acquired disturbances of thirst and vasopressin regulation). Klin. Wochenschr. **66** (1988) 498−501.

[19] Hensen, J., M. Dolz, W. Oelkers: Transiente Polyurie in der Schwangerschaft bei Diabetes insipidus und Gestationsdiabetes (Transient diabetes insipidus and diabetes mellitus in pregnancy). Med. Klin. **86** (1991) 623−628.

[20] Hensen, J. and P. Gross: Hypernatriämie und Diabetes insipidus. In: Gross, P. (ed.): Elektrolytstörungen in der Praxis, pp. 73−81. Programmed Verlag, Frankfurt 1991.

[21] Herzberg, N. H., E. Goudsmit, J. Kruisbrink et al.: Testosterone treatment restores reduced vasopressin-binding sites in the kidney of the aging rat. J. Endocrinol. **123** (1989) 59−63.

[22] Himmelstein, D. U., A. A. Jones, S. Woolhandler: Hypernatremic dehydration in nursing home patients: an indicator of neglect. J. Am. Geriatr. Soc. **31** (1983) 466−471.

[23] Jolkkonen, J., L. Tuomisto, T. B. Van Wimersma Greidanus et al.: Vasopressin levels in the cerebrospinal fluid in rats of different age and sex. Neuroendocrinology **44** (1986) 163−167.

[24] Kirkland, J., M. Lye, C. Goddard et al.: Plasma arginine vasopressin in dehydrated elderly patients. Clin. Endocrinol. (Oxf.) **20** (1984) 451−456.

[25] Lindeman, R. D., J. Tobin, N. W. Shock: Longitudinal studies on the rate of decline in renal function with age. J. Am. Geriatr. Soc. **33** (1985) 278−285.

[26] Lindeman, R. D., H. C. Van Buren, L. G. Raisz: Osmolar renal concentrating capacity in healthy young men and hospitalized patients without renal disease. N. Engl. J. Med. **262** (1960) 1306−1314.

[27] Ljungqvist, A., C. Lagergren: Normal intrarenal arterial pattern in adult and aging human kidney. J. Anat. **96** (1962) 285−300.

[28] McLean, K. A., P. A. O'Neill, I. Davies et al.: Influence of age on plasma osmolality: a community study. Age and Aging **21** (1992) 56−60.

[29] Miescher, E., S. M. Fortney: Responses to dehydration and rehydration during heat exposure in younger and older men. Am. J. Physiol. **257** (1989) R1050−R1056.

[30] Miller, J. H., N. W. Shock: Age differences in the renal tubular response to antidiuretic hormone. J. Gerontol. **8** (1953) 446−450.

[31] Miller, M.: Influence of aging on vasopressin secretion and water regulation. In: Schrier, R. W. (ed.): Vasopressin, pp. 249−258. Raven Press, New York 1985.

[32] Mooradian, A. D.: Water balance in the elderly. In: J. E. Morley, S. G. Korenman (eds.): Endocrinology and metabolism in the elderly, pp. 124−136. Blackwell Scientific Publications, Oxford 1992.

[33] O'Neill, P. A., E. B. Faragher, I. Davies et al.: Reduced survival with increasing plasma osmolality in elderly continuing-care patients − published erratum appears in Age Aging 1990 Sep; 19(5): 346−7 − see comments. Age and Aging **19** (1990) 68−71.

[34] Ohashi, M., N. Fujio, H. Nawata et al.: High plasma concentrations of human atrial natri-uretic polypeptide in aged man. J. Clin. Endocrinol. Metab. **64** (1987) 81−85.

[35] Phillips, P. A., M. Bretherton, C. I. Johnston et al.: Reduced osmotic thirst in healthy elderly men. Am. J. Physiol. Regul. Integr. Comp. Physiol. **261** (1991) R166−R171.

[36] Phillips, P. A., B. J. Rolls, J. G. G. Ledingham et al.: Reduced thirst after water deprivation in healthy elderly men. N. Engl. J. Med. **311** (1984) 753−759.

[37] Ravid, R., E. Fliers, D. F. Swaab et al.: Changes in vasopressin and testosterone in the senescent brown-Norway (BN/BiRij) rat. Gerontology **33** (1987) 87−98.

[38] Rondeau, E., J. deLima, H. Caillens et al.: High plasma antidiuretic hormone in patients with cardiac failure: Influence of age. Miner. Electrolyte Metab. **8** (1982) 267−274.

[39] Ross, E. J., S. B. M. Christie: Hypernatremia. Medicine **48** (1969) 441−473.

[40] Rowe, J. W., K. L. Minaker, D. Sparrow et al.: Age-related failure of volume-pressure-mediated vasopressin release. J. Clin. Endocrinol. Metab. **54** (1982) 661−664.

[41] Schoeller, D. A., Changes in total body water with age. Am. J. Clin. Nutr. **50** (1989) 1176−1181.

[42] Schrier, R. W., W. T. Abraham, J. Hensen: Strategies in management of acute renal failure in the intensive therapy unit. In: Bilhari, D., G. Neild (eds.): Acute renal failure in the intensive therapy unit, pp. 193−214. Springer Verlag, London−Berlin−New York 1990.

[43] Snyder, N. A., D. W. Feigal, A. I. Arieff: Hypernatremia in elderly patients. A heterogeneous, morbid, and iatrogenic entity. Ann. Intern. Med. **107** (1987) 309−319.

[44] Tryding, N., B. Berg, S. Ekman et al.: DDAVP test for renal concentration capacity. Age-related reference intervals. Cand. J. Urol. Nephrol. **22** (1988) 141−145.

[45] Yamamoto, T., H. Harada, J. Fukuyama et al.: Impaired arginine-vasopressin secretion associated with hypoangiotensinemia in hypernatremic dehydrated elderly patients. JAMA **259** (1988) 1039−1042.

[46] Zerbe, R. L., G. L. Robertson: Osmoregulation of thirst and vasopressin secretion in human subjects: effects of various solutes. Am. J. Physiol. **244** (1983) E607−E614.

The neuroendocrinology of the peri- and postmenopause

W. G. Rossmanith

1 Introduction

As a biological hallmark in the chronobiology of female life, the cessation of menstrual cyclicity during menopause indicates the end of reproductive capacity. A progressive decline in ovarian sex steroid release yields profound alterations in the neuroendocrine regulation of the reproductive system. An open-loop feedback system is created, comprised of the hypersecretion of gonadotropins from the pituitary in compensation for decreased secretion of ovarian sex steroids. This state of prolonged hypergonadotropic hypogonadism during the postmenopausal years may provide a unique model to delineate age-related alterations in the neuroendocrine control of reproductive hormone release. In particular, alterations in the hypothalamic and anterior pituitary function as neuroendocrine concomitants of aging may thus be discerned, prior to multiple pathologies known to occur at later stages of life [44]. By determining the changing gonadotropin dynamics during aging in postmenopausal women, several questions can be addressed. As yet, the principal sites of aging in endocrine systems are still ill defined. More specifically, uncertainty exists as to whether aging involves a hypothalamic decline rather than a pituitary hypofunction [40]. Further, the sensitivity of the central regulatory units to sex steroid feedback may be severely affected by age [38]. Central neurotransmitter activity implicated in the control of gonadotropin release may also be altered [15].

To address some mechanisms presumed to be involved in the process of neuroendocrine aging, we have aimed to determine the serum gonadotropin pulsatility during the aging process in postmenopausal women. Based on the demonstration of close functional and temporal links between hypothalamic signals and pituitary gonadotropin release [2, 14], this approach of evaluating age-related processes in humans appears to be justified. Changes in the serum gonadotropin profiles may thus reflect altered neuroendocrine functions with advancing age in postmenopausal women. In addition, determination of the gonadotropin-releasing hormone (GnRH)-stimulated gonadotropin secretion can serve as a useful parameter to discern age-related hyopthalamic effects from those of the pituitary.

In this chapter, the LH pulsatile secretion of peri- and postmenopausal women will be characterized as an unrestrained rhythm, reflecting the maximum activity of the central "pulse generator" [3, 10]. Alterations in the gonadotropin secretion of aged women will then be related to this basal pulsatility. In particular, eventual alterations in the feedback sensitivity and neurotransmitter control of gonadotropin release will be explored. Most presented evidence for neuroendocrine age-associated processes is based on recent investigations involving pre- and postmenopausal women. Secretory dynamics so determined during aging in humans may collectively reflect the cumulative alterations in the neuroendocrine mechanisms governing gonadotropin release. The presented findings will provide detailed insight into the neuroendocrine concomitants of aging in women. Effort has been made to focus primarily on observations in humans, but results obtained from experimental animals were also considered for a meaningful interpretation. Many important findings on the age-related endocrine alterations in humans and animals can be only incompletely appreciated in this brief essay. Therefore, several extended reviews are recommended for a more comprehensive analysis [15, 16, 19, 35, 38, 45].

2 Hypotheses of aging

During the past two decades, our understanding of the neuroendocrine processes of aging has been considerably enlarged. Results from recent investigations towards the exploration of neuronal processes involved in aging [19, 38] have attracted increasing interest in this research area. Endocrine functions exhibit a decline very early in life. Although several neuroendocrine alterations are observed during menopause, they may just coincidentally be related to this period. Results from studies during peri- and postmenopause may in fact represent functional alterations which already originated much earlier in life [16]. Evidence has now accumulated to suggest that neuroendocrine aging may precipitate changes in the interrelationship between hormonal and neural signals rather than being isolated neuroendocrine events [40].

Since the early investigations, several theories of endocrine aging have been proposed. Intrinsic or extrinsic influences [5, 15, 40] have been implicated as biological requirements for aging systems. Furthermore, a classical hypothesis is that biological aging represents the lifetime accumulation of environmental insults and errors in cell reduplication [5, 40]. Another theory is based on the suggestion that aging relates to genetically predetermined events that are critical for the survival of the species [5]. Experimental evidence does not sufficiently support any of these assumptions, and none of them have been conclusively proven. However, these theories may help to develop a general concept of sites and mechanisms involved in the neuroendocrinology of the aging reproductive system.

3 Characterization of ultradian and circadian variations in the LH pulsatility of postmenopausal women

Secretion of gonadotropins is invariably increased in postmenopausal women [5, 28, 31, 46−48]. Since any considerable negative feedback exerted by ovarian sex steroid on the hypothalamic-pituitary system is absent in postmenopausal women [25, 48], their gonadotropin release is enhanced as consequence of an open feedback loop. During the perimenopausal period, concentrations of follicle-stimulating hormone (FSH) rise initially, followed by a gradual increase in luteinizing hormone (LH) levels [5, 8, 46]. The secretion of gonadotropins has been demonstrated to be episodic ("pulsatile") in nature [10, 25, 46, 47]. In fact, these LH pulse characteristics become very prominent in women after menopause, compared to normally cycling women (Fig. 1a). Since the gonadotropin secretion patterns of postmenopausal women are virtually unmodulated by ovarian sex steroid influence [25, 27], the pulse attributes of this basic rhythm may reflect the maximum activity of the central pulse generator [25, 31].

In the LH secretory profiles of postmenopausal women, the pulses are set at frequencies similar to those seen in normally cycling women, albeit with much higher pulse amplitudes (Fig. 1a). That the LH pulsatility during postmenopause indeed represents the maximum release rates of the central GnRH-LH pace-maker, is evidenced by the finding that increases and decreases in the LH pulse attributes in women during the menstrual cycle are limited by the pulse characteristics of postmenopausal subjects (Fig. 1b). Thus, the LH pulse frequencies and amplitudes of postmenopausal women indicate a threshold, which the changing LH pulse attributes during the menstrual cycle never exceed [25, 31]. Even during periods of increasing serum concentrations of sex steorids as during the menstrual cycle including the midcycle LH surge, the LH pulse attributes can just approximate those of postmenopausal women. Collectively, the LH pulsatility of hypogonadal postmenopausal women reflects the activity of a spontaneously depolarizing system at its maximum rate [31].

In the presence of the remaining serum androgen concentrations, this basic pulse rhythm is not restrained. Androgen receptor blockage fails to noticeably modify the LH pulsatility of postmenopausal women [26]. Likewise, the changing LH pulsatility during ovarian sex steroid replacement in postmenopausal women is also confined to the pulse attributes of the unrestrained LH rhythm during unreplaced conditions. While exposure to estrogen clearly suppresses the mean LH secretion (Fig. 2a), it does not noticeably enhance the LH frequencies and amplitudes. Conversely, progesterone administration markedly slows the frequencies (Fig. 2b). As a consequence, the changes in the LH pulsatile attributes during a high sex steroid exposure, as during the menstrual cycle or

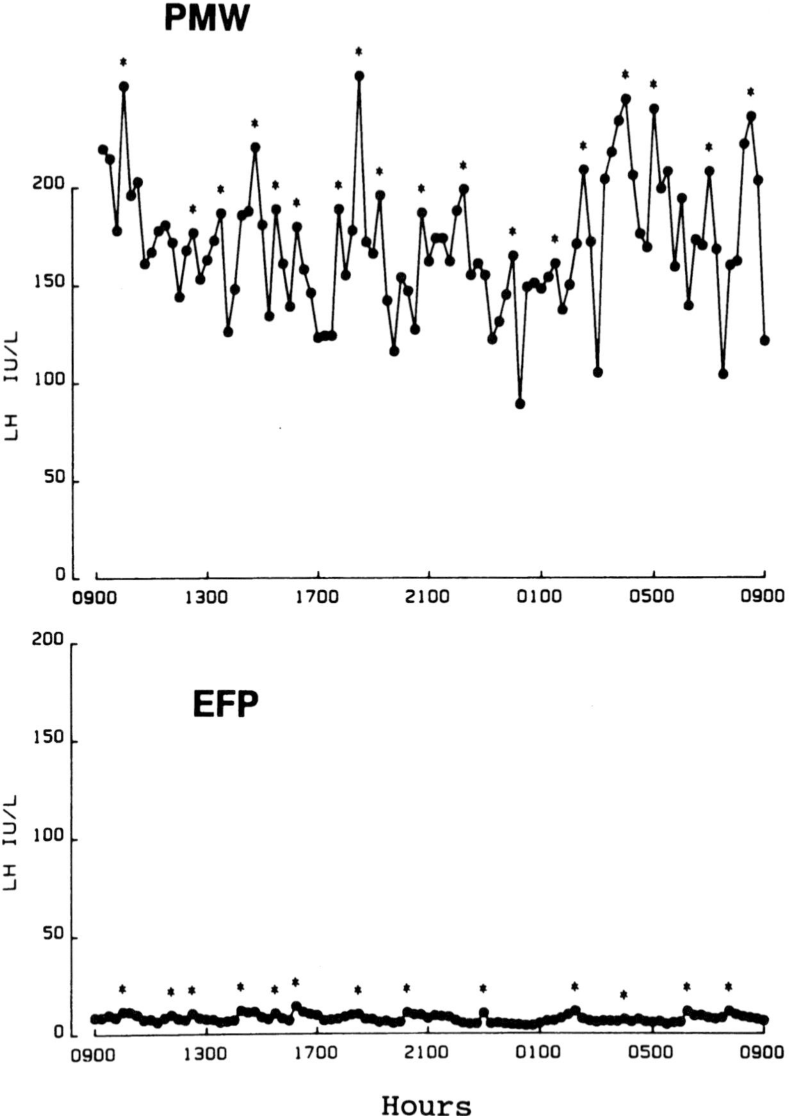

Fig. 1a   24-hour LH secretory profiles in a woman during postmenopause (PMW, top) and in a woman during the early follicular phase of her cycle (EFP, bottom). Asterisks indicate significant pulses.

during hormone replacement in hypogonadal states, are confined to the characteristics of the unrestrained pulsatility of postmenopausal women [31].

Moreover, gonadotropin release in postmenopausal women is characterized by circadian variabilities on which the gonadotropin secretory episodes are super-

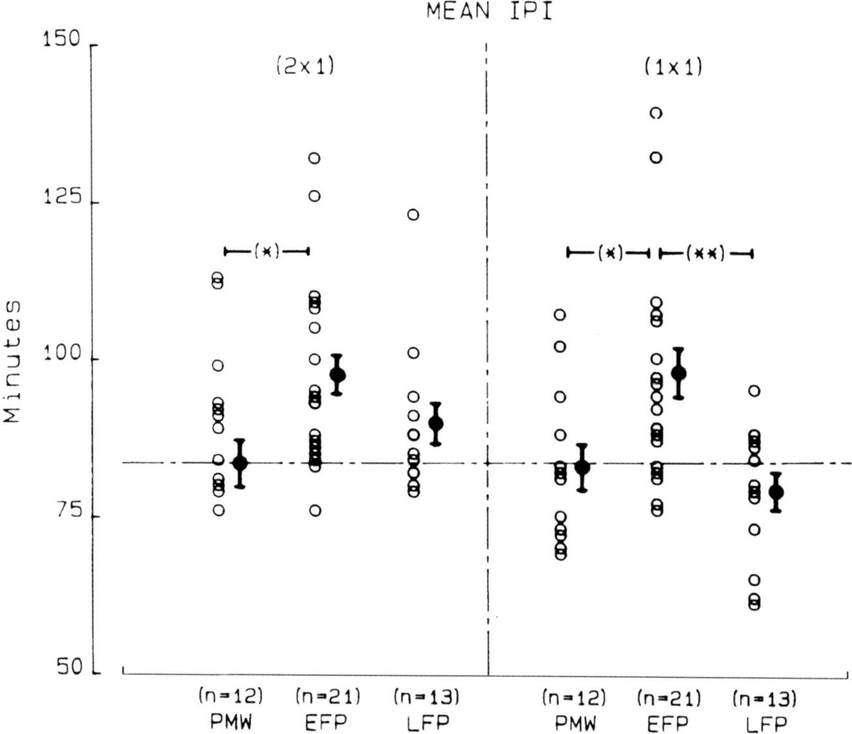

Fig. 1b Individual interpulse intervals determined in the 24-hour LH secretory profiles of postmenopausal women (PMW) and in women during the early follicular phase (EFP) and late follicular phase (LFP) of their cycles. Interpulse intervals were identified by the Cluster pulse algorithm using two different cluster sizes. The symbols bordering the individual data represent the mean ± SEM. * p < 0.05, ** p < 0.01 compared with values linked with brackets.

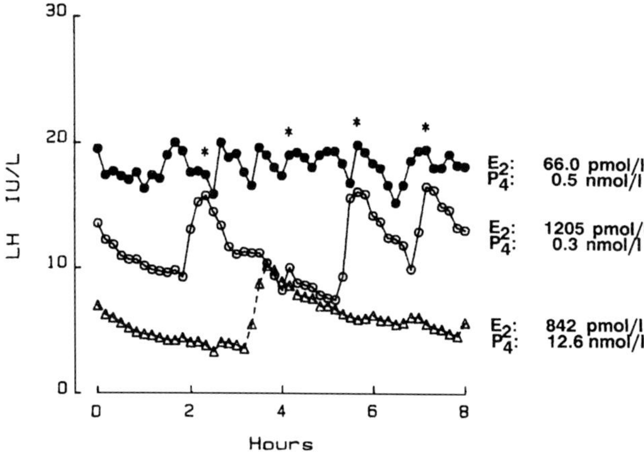

Fig. 2a LH secretory profiles of a postmenopausal women before (closed circles) and during E_2 (open circles) or E_2/P_4 replacement therapies (open triangles). Asterisks indicate significant pulses.

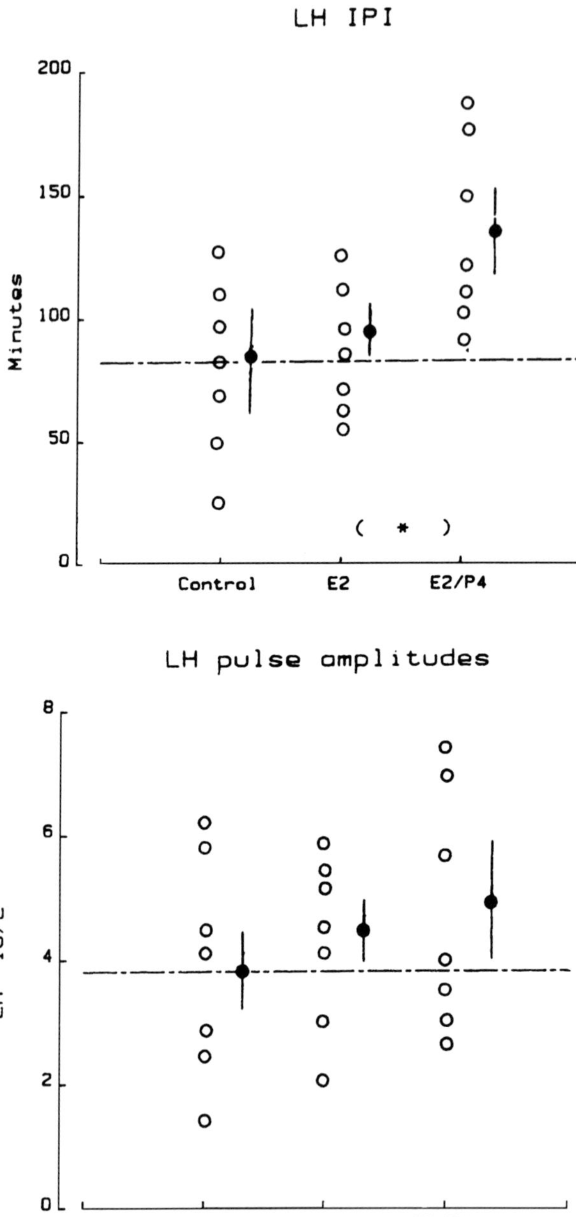

Fig. 2b   Individual and mean ($\pm$ SEM) LH interpulse intervals and pulse amplitudes of seven post-menopausal women before replacement (= control) and during E_2 or E_2/P_4 replacement regimens. The horizontal line indicates the mean values during control conditions. * $p < 0.05$ vs. values linked with brackets.

imposed [20, 28]. A circadian rhythm was not only disclosed for the mean gonadotropin secretion rates, but also for the magnitudes of the pulse attributes [28]. The characteristics of these circadian swings vary in accordance with the prevailing sex steroid milieu, and thus differ in postmenopausal and normally cycling women [20, 28]. In postmenopausal women, highest LH pulse amplitudes are found during the night hours, at about the time when maximal LH secretion is attained [28]. The preservation of a circadian clock in the LH pulsatile secretion during the years of early postmenopauses is in keeping with the notion that the endocrine system remains responsive despite advancement of age [40]. As it appears, a diurnal variability in the gonadotropin secretion may pertain to the time of senescence in women [6], although subtle time-shifts or an attenuation of this rhythmicity cannot be excluded in the elderly women. Age-related alterations in the circadian variability of hormone release have been proposed to subserve a deficit in physiological endocrine performance [40].

4 Gonadotropin secretion during aging in postmenopausal women

In the years during and after menopause, gonadotropin levels considerably increase [8, 25, 47, 48]. While aging progresses in postmenopause, gonadotropin secretion gradually declines, so that the gonadotropin levels during senescence almost approximate those of the premenopausal period [27]. Fewer LH and FSH secretory episodes with lower pulse amplitudes are observed in aged women, compared with postmenopausal women during their first decade after natural onset of menopause (Fig. 3). Since the metabolic clearance rates of gonadotropins remain virtually unaffected by age [11], this attenuated gonadotropin pulsatility of older postmenopausal women may indeed relate to a declined gonadotropin release from the pituitary. However, the gonadotropin pulse frequencies primarily reflect the intermittent pituitary activation by episodic GnRH release [10, 48]. Therefore, the finding of lower gonadotropin pulse frequencies in aged postmenopausal women permit us to infer that the reduced gonadotropin secretion in old age may relate to a functional decline in the hypothalamic GnRH pulse generator, although a pituitary site of action cannot be entirely excluded [27]. This notion is further substantiated by the finding of a progressive loss of GnRH neurons at various hypothalamic sites [45]. Moreover, the GnRH content of the hypothalamus has been reported to decrease with advanced age in humans [21] and in experimental animals [16]. This age-related deficit in GnRH release can effectively be restored in the old female rat, so that estrous cyclicity is resumed [16]. This finding clearly indicates a hypothalamic site as principal cause of the age-related attenuation in gonado-

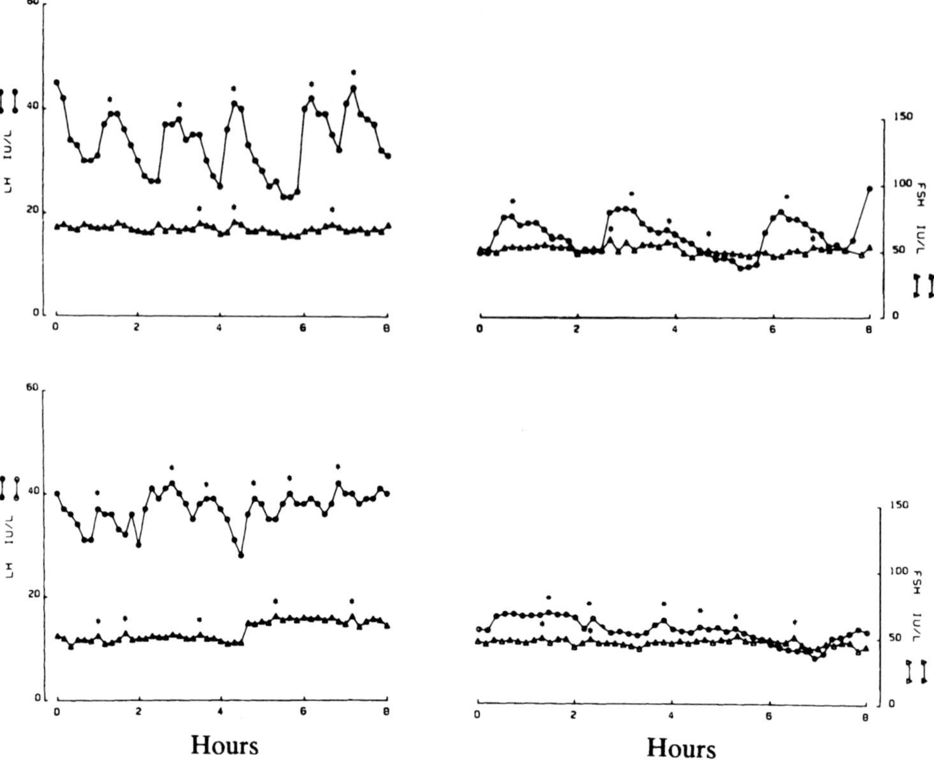

Fig. 3   Representative LH (circles) and FSH (triangles) secretory profiles of two younger (left) and two older postmenopausal women. Asterisks indicate significant pulses (from [27]).

tropin secretion. Prolonged estrogen exposure has been demonstrated to decrease the number of functioning of hypothalamic GnRH neurons [1, 4], suggesting a pivotal role for ovarian sex steroids in the hypothalamic processes of aging.

The observation of a decreased gonadotropin release in postmenopausal women is in keeping with previous results of some [8, 27], but not all investigations conducted [5, 33]. The differences may at least partially be reconciled by the heterogeneity of the studied populations. It is well established that concurrent endocrinological and general illnesses interfere with gonadotropin secretion in postmenopausal women [19]. Therefore, results obtained in affected women need to be carefully excluded from analysis, not to confound the interpretation. Moreover, the validity of single hormone determinations as performed in earlier studies may be questioned, in view of the marked differences between nadir and peak hormone concentrations [27].

5 Is pituitary gonadotropin responsiveness preserved during aging in postmenopausal women?

It has been proposed that the GnRH-stimulated gonadotropin response is clearly exaggerated in postmenopausal subjects, compared to premenopausal women [33, 41]. We have conducted our investigation in a large cohort of pre- and postmenopausal women to determine the effects, if any, of advancing age on pituitary gonadotropin responsiveness. GnRH was found to stimulate the LH and FSH secretion during different stages of life in women (Fig. 4). The absolute gonadotropin release following GnRH stimulations was determined to be highest in postmenopausal women. However, when the percentage gonadotropin increments were considered to take variances in the basal gonadotropin concentrations into account, these differences no longer existed. Thus, the pituitary gonadotroph resopnsiveness is preserved with progressive aging in women. In particular, it does not vary between postmenopausal women of different ages [29]. Despite the prolonged exposure to low estrogen levels and the high rates of gonadotropin secretion in postmenopause, the pituitary release capacity is apparently not impaired in older women. While earlier studies have claimed a decreased gonadotropin release in response to GnRH stimulations in elderly subjects [8], the findings of the current and other investigations [7, 33] challenge this notion. Results in experimental animals also suggest no considerable age-releated deficit in the pituitary function. Pituitary transplants from aged into younger female rats effectively maintained estrous cyclicity [15]. Aging was also not associated with a decline in pituitary GnRH receptor density [37]. Collectively, these results suggest that pituitary gonadotropin responsiveness is preserved in old age, further stressing the importance of a hypothalamic functional decline as the principal mechanism for the age-related attenuation of gonadotropin secretion in women.

However, it should be noted that quantitative changes in the pituitary hormones may also occur during aging [43]. The physico-chemical characteristics of the gonadotropin molecular moieties show a polymorphism with aging in humans. Large LH forms display slower metabolic rates and different biological profiles than the minor ones [39]. As deduced from our gonadotropin determinations obtained by radioimmunoassay measurements (Fig. 4), the gonadotropins may be released in response to GnRH stimulations at fairly constant rates throughout pre- and postmenopausal life. Yet, the biological potency of these GnRH-stimulated gonadotropins may vary with the advance of age, as a result of different distribution patterns in the gonadotropin moieties.

6 Can feedback actions by ovarian sex steroids still be activated in elderly postmenopausal women?

It is well established that ovarian sex steriod replacement decreases both the LH and FSH levels in postmenopausal women [38, 41]. Since FSH is more sensitive to the negative feedback effects of estrogen than LH [48], other factors than changes in hypothalamic GnRH release are assumed to account for the differential suppression of these gonadotropins. Estradiol replacement in post-menopausal women does not completely return the FSH serum levels to normal, indicating that additional regulatory components, such as ovarian inhibin, may play a major role in feedback regulation [19]. Early studies suggested that post-menopausal women may be more responsive to estrogen negative feedback than

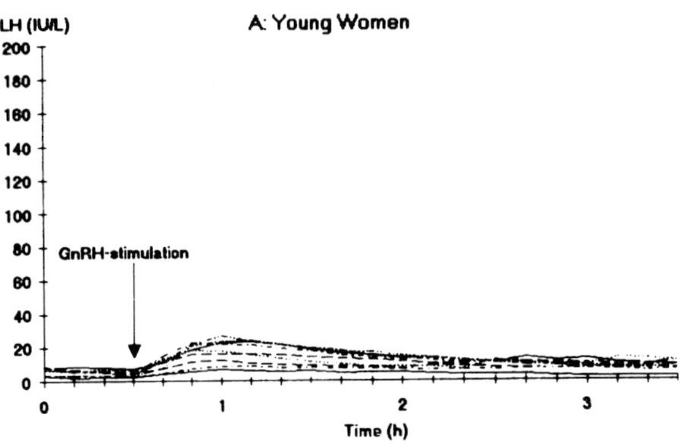

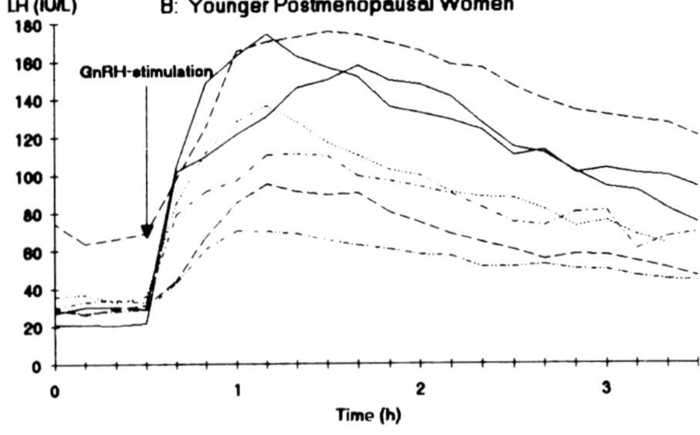

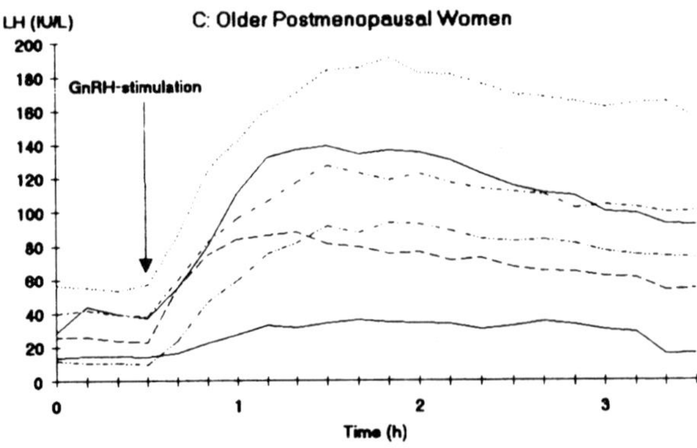

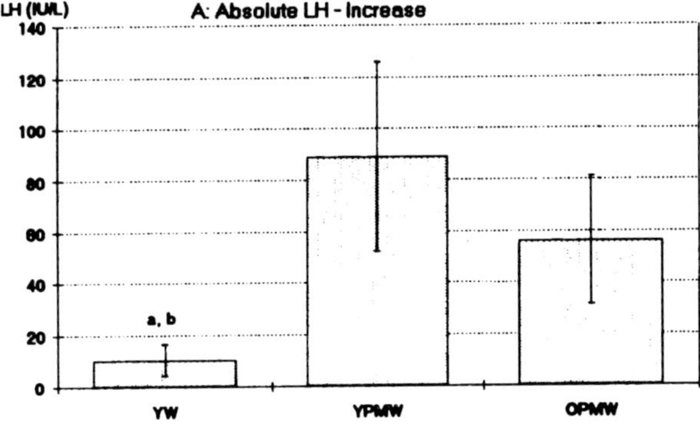

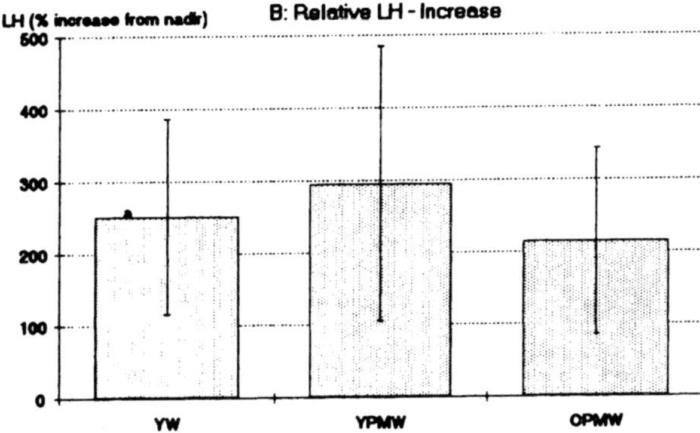

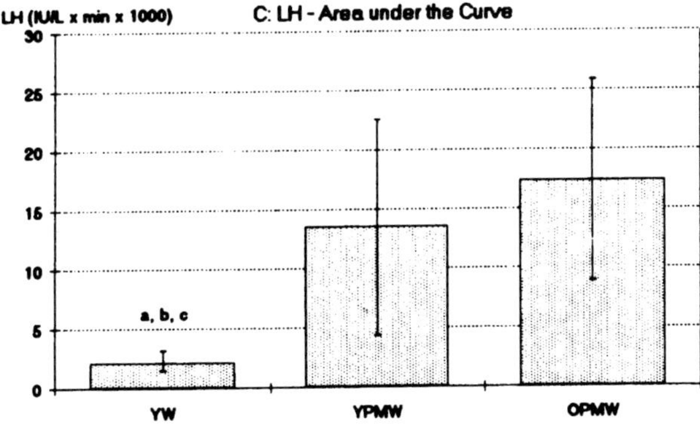

Fig. 4 Individual LH responses to GnRH stimulations (25 μg i. v., Fig. 5a) and absolute and relative LH increments (Fig. 5b) in nine younger women (mean age: 25.6 years), seven younger (mean age: 56.6 years) and six older postmenopausal women (mean age: 81.9 years). YW, young women; YPMW, younger postmenopausal women; OPMW, older postmenopausal women. a = p < 9.01 vs. values of younger PMW, b = p < 0.05 vs. values of older PMW.

premenopausal subjects [41]. However, this assumption has been questioned, based on the marked differences in the experimental methodologies [5].

Whether the negative feedback sensitivity of gonadotropins to sex steroid exposure may pertain to postmenopausal women of advanced age remains unresolved.

Accordingly, we have used the anti-estrogen clomiphene citrate to probe the gonadotropin sensitivity to negative feedback in postmenopausal women of different ages [30]. During the low estrogen milieu of postmenopause, the anti-estrogen is virtually recognized as estrogenic compound [48]. Similar to the gonadotropin suppression previously noted during estradiol replacement therapies [Fig. 2a], clomiphene citrate may act to attenuate the gonadotropin secretion in postmenopausal women. In fact, when clomiphene citrate was administered to postmenopausal women during the first decade after the onset of meno-

Younger postmenopausal woman

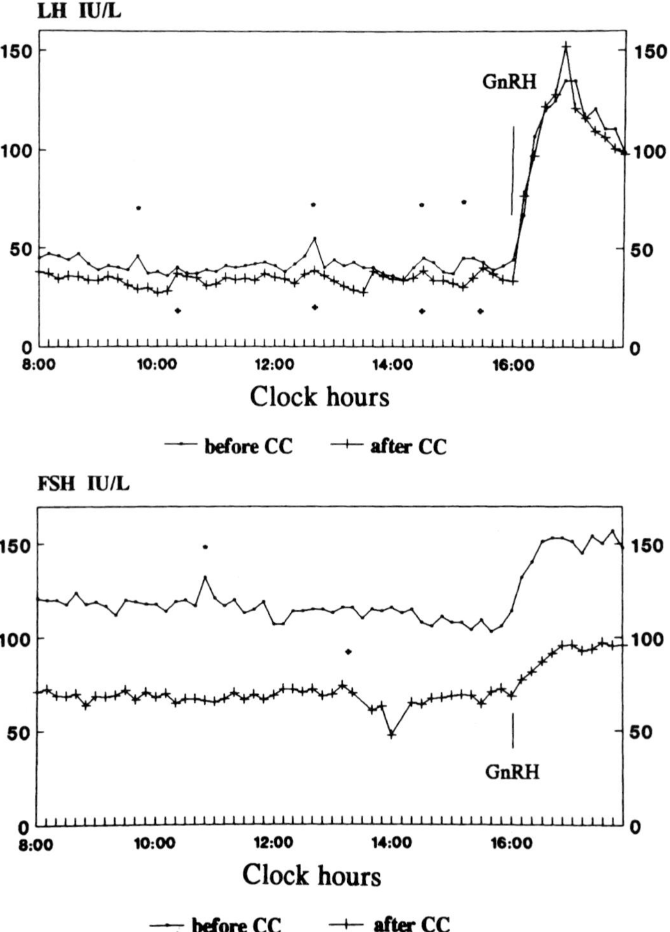

Older postmenopausal woman

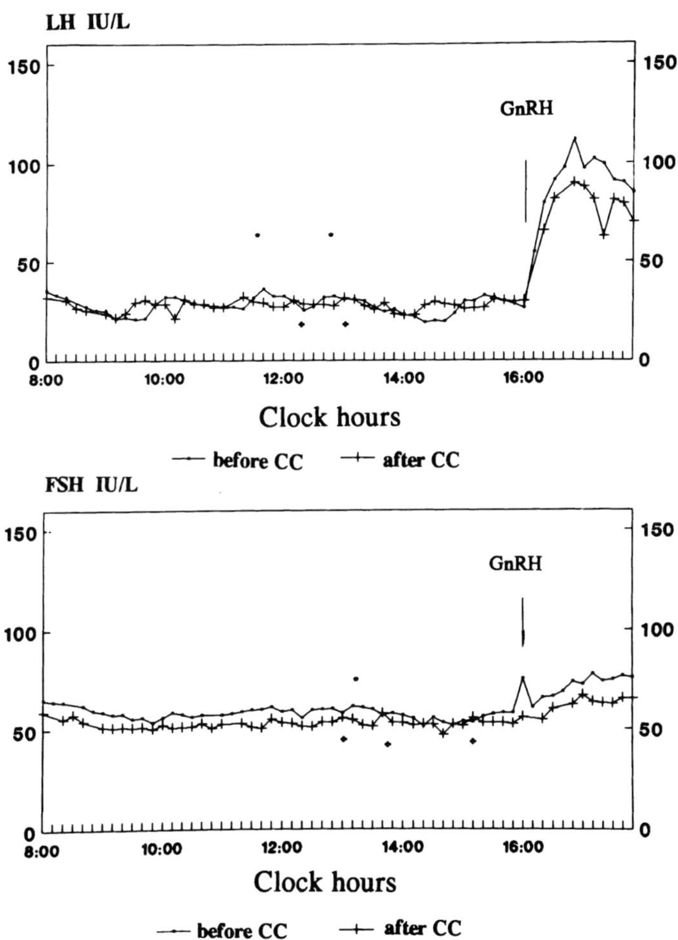

Fig. 5   Unstimulated and GnRH-stimulated LH and FSH secretory profiles of a younger and an older postmenopausal woman before and during administration of clomiphene citrate (CC). Asteriks indicate significant pulses.

pause, the pulsatile LH and FSH release was found to be markedly suppressed (Fig. 5). these observations favor the concept that the sensitivity of the hypothalamic-pituitary unit to negative feedback may be preserved during the early years of postmenopause [30]. In contrast, no such changes in the pulsatile gonadotropin release were noted in elderly postmenopausal women, and their pituitary responsiveness remained unaffected by anti-estrogen administration. Therefore, the sensitivity to negative feedback exerted by ovarian sex steroids may be attenuated or even completely lost as aging progresses in postmenopausal women. This finding apparently relates to hypothalamic defects rather than to a pituitary functional deficit [30]. Recent findings in rodents have suggested an age-associated decline in the sensitivity of the hypothalamus to hormonal feedback [40]. Indeed, an increased hypothalamic threshold to negative sex steroid feedback has been noted in old rats [34]. Aging may therefore precipitate a shift in the sensitivity of the hypothalamus to specific hormone actions. Conversely, processes of aging presumably comprise a discordant pattern of sensitivity changes, during which some of the nuclei become more and others less sensitive to negative hormonal signals [40].

Feedback effects of the anti-estrogen clomiphene citrate on the hypothalamic-pituitary unit have also been evaluated in aging men. Irrespective of their age, their gonadotropin pulsatility was found to be markedly influenced in response to administration of anti-estrogen. Combined with our observation of a loss of feedback sensitivity in old postmenopausal women, these findings suggest a sex dimorphism in the age-related development of the negative feedback control. Relevant to this concept may be the observation that testosterone protects the GnRH containing neuronal system from a numeric and functional decay during biological aging, while prolonged estrogen exposure facilitates the loss of hypothalamic neurons [4].

High doses of estradiol may also induce a positive feedback effect on gonadotropin secretion in postmenopausal women. A surge-like increase could be elicited by exposing peri- and postmenopausal women to increasing concentrations of estrogen [9, 48]. Whether such positive feedback on gonadotropin secretion can also be evoked in older postmenopausal women awaits further clarification.

7 Neurotransmitter activity on gonadotropin secretion during aging in postmenopausal women

An imbalanced neurotransmitter control of gonadotropin secretion has been implicated as a possible explanation for age-related functional alterations. As inferred from the animal model, the hormonal changes with aging may not result from a complete loss of transmitter activity, but rather relate to a desynchronization and disorganization of the interrelated neuronal and endocrine signals [40]. Advancement of age does not only influence the effective concentrations of classical neurotransmitters at their target sites in the brain, but may also affect the receptor density and the affinity of neurotransmitters to bind to their receptors [15, 42].

Current evidence, although still anecdotal, suggests a decreased functioning of the monoaminergic neuronal system in humans [15, 40]. Our evaluation of the dopaminergic inhibition on gonadotropin secretion indicates a marked impairment of the central dopaminergic activity in postmenopausal women [24]. In fact, use of a dopamine receptor blocker fails to significantly modify the gonadotropin secretory patterns of postmenopausal women. To our knowledge, there are no studies which critically address the eventual restoration of dopaminergic inhibitory tone following sex steroid replacement in postmenopausal women. Conversely, the gonadotropin secretion of postmenopausal women could effectively be suppressed by administration of dopamine or its agonists [12, 13]. It is therefore suggested that the attenuated dopaminergic activity on gonadotropin secretion found after onset of menopause may relate, among other determinants, to changes in the number and affinity of dopaminergic receptors [42]. Monoaminergic production rates decline as aging progresses in experimental animals [16, 44]. Profound alteration has been found for the dopaminergic content in the mediobasal hypothalamus [16, 40] and for the dopamine concentrations in the hypothalamic-pituitary portal system of old rats [36]. Thus, we propose that decreased central dopaminergic activity may facilitate a self-destruction process, with further derangements in the endocrine homeostasis during senescence in women [5].

The enhanced gonadotropin levels during postmenopause have been attributed, in addition to other factors, to a decline in opioidergic inhibition on GnRH-LH secretion. Endogenous opioid activity is absent in postmenopausal women [22, 32], but opioidergic inhibition can effectively be restored by estrogen replacement in postmenopausal women [17]. In turn, dopaminergic activity may mediate some of the effects of endogenous opioid tone, since administration of a dopamine agonist to postmenopausal women successfully re-installs the opioidergic inhibition on gonadotropin release [18]. Collectively, these findings indicate close functional links between the opioidergic and dopaminergic neuronal systems in postmenopausal women [32]. Thus, combined alterations in the central dopaminergic [23, 36], opioidergic [17] and serotoninergic pathways [5, 38] may subserve the age-related alterations found in the gonadotropin release of postmenopausal women. Whether derangements in the neurotransmitter activity continue to progress and then account for the profound attenuation of gonadotropin secretion in old postmenopausal women still remains to be elucidated.

8 Conclusions

Evidence provided by the current and several other investigations has accumulated to suggest that biological aging during postmenopause markedly affects the neuroendocrine system governing gonadotropin release. The presented studies and their interpretations may be important to expand our knowledge of the neuroendocrine age-related processes. The determination of changing secretory dynamics in the gonadotropin secretion of postmenopausal women proves to be a valid approach to delineate alterations as a function of progressing age. Hence, a putative model is proposed, highlighting the potential sites of alterations in the hypothalamic-pituitary system with advancing age in

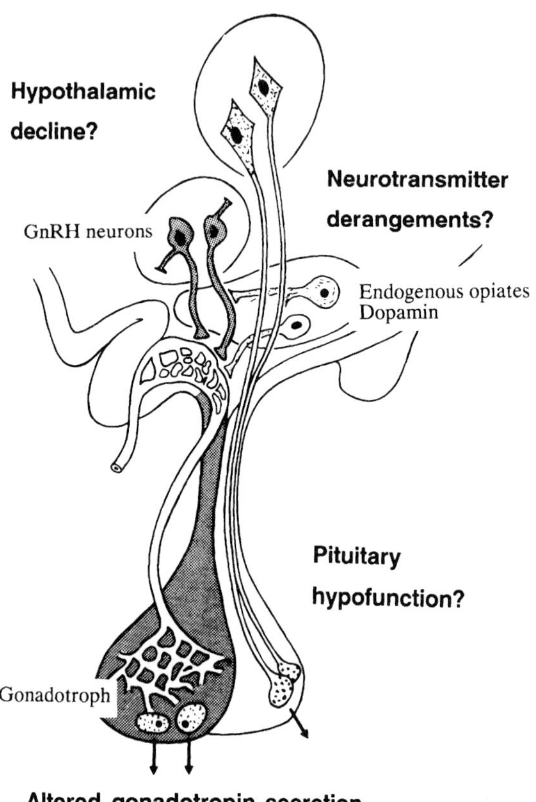

Fig. 6 Schematic representation of the putative central target sites involved in the processes of aging in humans.

humans (Fig. 6). In this simplified concept, major functional deficits, primarily at a hypothalamic rather than a pituitary site, have been delineated as concomitants of aging in women. Moreover, aging may also impair the negative feedback sensitivity to ovarian sex steorids, and derangements in the central neurotransmitter activity may run parallel to this decline. By appraising the physiological meaning of the presented findings, we are tempted to propose that the process of aging relates to a hypothalamic decline rather than to a pituitary hypofunction.

Albeit considerably advanced, our current understanding of the neuroendocrine processes during aging in humans still remains inconclusive. More detailed insights into the complex neuroendocrine alterations during aging may provide better methodologies for the appropriate prevention or attenuation of deleterious effects by specific interventions [40].

Acknowledgements

The author wishes to express his gratitude to Drs. C. Lauritzen, W. A. Scherbaum and S. S. C. Yen for their support in completion of the studies, and to Dr. Benz, Dr. Handke-Vesely, M. Beuter, S. Schurer, C. Reichelt and B. Lüttke for their technical assistance. W. G. R. is recipient of Deutsche Forschungsgemeinschaft grants (DFG Ro 657/2-1 and 3-1).

References

[1] Brawer, J. R., H. Schipper, F. Naftolin: Ovary-dependent degeneration in the hypothalamic arcuate nucleus. Endocrinology 107 (1980) 274–279.

[2] Clarke, I. J., J. T. Cummins: The temporal relationship between gonadotropin-releasing hormone (GnRH) and luteinizing hormone (LH) secretion in ovariectomized ewes. Endocrinology 111 (1982) 1737–1739.

[3] Dyer, R. G., J. E. Robinson: The LHRH pulse generator. J. Endocrinol. 123 (1989) 1–2.

[4] Finch, C. E., C. V. Mobbs: Hormonal influences on hypothalamic sensitivity during aging in female rodents. In: J. Meites (ed.): Neuroendocrinology of Aging, pp. 143–171. Plenum Press, New York 1983.

[5] Hammond, C. B., S. J. Ory: Endocrine aspects of the menopause. In: R. P. Sherman (ed.): Clinical Reproductive Endocrinology, pp. 185–194. Livingstone, New York 1985.

[6] Haus, E., G. Nicolau, D. J. Lakatau et al.: Circadian rhythm parameters of endocrine functions in elderly subjects during the seventh to the ninth decade of life. Chronobiologia 16 (1989) 331–352.

[7] Hanker, J. P., U. Ende, H. G. Bohnet et al.: Intermittent stimulation with LH-RH in postmenopausal hypergonadotropinism. Horm. Metab. Res. 13 (1981) 696–699.

[8] Judd, J. W. W., W. P. Collins, J. D. Forecast et al.: Plasma hormone profiles after the menopause and bilateral oophorectomy. Postgrad. Med. J. 54 (1978) 25–30.

[9] Kempers, R. D., R. J. Ryan: Acute effects of intravenous infusion of 17β-estradiol and 17α-hydroxyprogesterone on gonadotropin release. Fertil. Steril. 28 (1977) 631–635.

[10] Knobil, E.: The neuroendocrine control of the menstrual cycle. Rec. Prog. Horm. Res. 36 (1980) 53–88.

[11] Kohler, P. O., G. T. Ross, W. D. O'Dell: Metabolic clearance and production rates of human luteinizing hormone in pre- and postmenopausal women. J. Clin. Invest. 47 (1968) 38–47.

[12] Lachelin, G. C. L., H. Leblanc, S. S. C. Yen: The inhibitory effects of dopamine agonists on LH release in women. J. Clin. Endocrinol. Metab. 44 (1977) 728–732.

[13] Leblanc, H., G. C. L. Lachelin, S. Abu-Fadil et al.: Effects of dopamine infusion on pituitary hormone secretion in humans. J. Clin. Endocrinol. Metab. 43 (1976) 668–674.

[14] Levine, J. E., R. L. Norman, P. M. Gliessman et al.: In vivo gonadotropin-releasing hormone release and serum luteinizing hormone measurements in ovariectomized, estrogen-treated rhesus monkeys. Endocrinology **117** (1985) 711—721.

[15] Meites, J., H. H. Huang, J. W. Simpkins et al.: Central nervous system neurotransmitters during the decline of reproductive activity. In: P. Fioretti, L. Martini, G. B. Melis et al. (eds.): The Menopause: Clinical, Endocrinological and Pathophysiological Aspects, pp. 3—14. Academic Press, London 1982.

[16] Meites, J.: Alterations in hypothalamic-pituitary function with age. In: H. J. Armbrecht, R. M. Coe, N. Wongsurawat (eds.): Endocrine Function and Aging, pp. 1—12. Springer, New York 1988.

[17] Melis, G. B., A. Cagnacci, M. Gambacciani et al.: Chronic bromocryptine administration restores luteinizing hormone response to naloxone in postmenopausal women. Neuroendocrinology **47** (1988) 159—163.

[18] Melis, G. B., A. M. Paoletti, M. Gambacciani et al.: Evidence that estrogens inhibit LH secretion through opioids in postmenopausal women using naloxone. Neuroendocrinology **39** (1984) 60—63.

[19] Morley, J. E., S. G. Korenman, F. E. Kaiser: The menopause. In: J. E. Morley, S. G. Korenman (eds.): Endocrinology and Metabolism in the Elderly, pp. 322—335. Blackwell Scientific Publications, Oxford 1992.

[20] Mortola, J. F., G. A. Laughlin, S. S. C. Yen: A circadian rhythm of serum follicle-stimulating hormone in women. J. Clin. Endocrinol. Metab. **75** (1992) 861—864.

[21] Parker, C. R., J: C. Porter: Luteinizing hormone-releasing hormone and thyrotropin-releasing hormone in the hypothalamus of women: effects of age and reproductive status. J. Clin. Endocrinol. Metab. **58** (1984) 488—491.

[22] Reid, R. L., M. E. Quigley, S. S. C. Yen: The disappearance of opioidergic regulation of gonadotropin secretion in postmenopausal women. J. Clin. Endocrinol. Metab. **57** (1983) 1107—1110.

[23] Reymond, M. J., A. Donda, T. Lemarchand-Bèraud: Neuroendocrine aspects of aging: experimental data. Horm. Res. **31** (1989) 32—38.

[24] Rossmanith, W. G., U. Wirth, S. S. C. Yen: Does prolonged dopaminergic blockade alter the LH pulsatile secretion in normal cycling and postmenopausal women? Acta Endocrinol. **121** (1989) 147—152.

[25] Rossmanith, W. G., C. H. Liu, G. A. Laughlin et al.: Relative changes in LH pulsatility during the menstrual cycle: using data from hypogonadal women as a reference point. Clin. Endocrinol. **32** (1990) 647—660.

[26] Rossmanith, W. G., M. Beuter, R. Benz et al.: How do androgens affect the episodic gonadotrophin secretion in postmenopausal women? Maturitas **13** (1991) 325—335.

[27] Rossmanith, W. G., W. A. Scherbaum, C. Lauritzen: Gonadotropin secretion during aging in postmenopausal women. Neuroendocrinology **54** (1991) 211—218.

[28] Rossmanith, W. G., C. Lauritzen: The luteinizing hormone pulsatile secretion: circadian excursion in eugonadal and hypogonadal women. Gynecol. Endocrinol. **54** (1991) 249—265.

[29] Rossmanith, W. G., B. Lüttke, R. Benz et al.: Gonadotropin responsiveness during aging in men and women. Proceedings of the Symposion on Gonadotropins, GnRH, GnRH analogs and Gonadal Peptides. Paris 1992.

[30] Rossmanith, W. G., C. Reichelt, R. Benz et al.: Effects of clomiphene citrate on the gonadotropin secretion in postmenopausal women of different age. Proceedings of the Symposion on Gonadotropins, GnRH, GnRH analogs and Gonadal Peptides. Paris 1992.

[31] Rossmanith, W. G.: Circulating luteinizing hormone (LH) patterns during female reproductive life. In: A. R. Genazzani, F. Petraglia (eds.): Hormones in Gynecological Endocrinology, pp. 225—240. Parthenon Publishing, Carnforth 1992.

[32] Rossmanith, W. G.: Endogenous opioid regulation of luteinizing hormone (LH) secretion in women. In: M. Negri, G. Lotti, A. Grossman (eds.): Clinical Perspectives of Opioid Peptide Production, pp. 134–159. Wiley and Sons, London 1992.

[33] Scaglia, H., M. Medina, A. L. Pinto-Ferreira et al.: Pituitary LH and FSH secretion and responsiveness in women of old age. Acta Endocrinol. 81 (1976) 673–679.

[34] Shaar, C. J., J. S. Euker, G. D. Riegle et al.: Effects of castration and gonadal steroids on serum LH and prolactin in old and young rats. J. Endocrinol. 66 (1975) 45–51.

[35] Simpkins, J. W., W. J. Millard: Influence of age on neurotransmitter function. In: B. Sacktor (ed.): Endocrinology and Aging. Endocrinology and Metabolism Clinics of North America, pp. 893–917. Saunders, Philadelphia 1987.

[36] Simpkins, J. W., G. P. Mueller, H. H. Huang et al.: Evidence for depressed catecholamine and enhanced serotonin metabolism in aging male rats: possible relation to gonadotropin secretion. Endocrinology 100 (1977) 1672–1678.

[37] Sonntag, W., J. Forman, J. Fiori: Decreased ability of old male rats to secrete luteinizing hormone (LH) is not due to alterations in pituitary LH-releasing hormone receptors. Endocrinology 114 (1984) 1657–1664.

[38] Steger, R. W., J. J. Peluso: Sex hormones in the aging female. In: B. Sacktor (ed.): Endocrinology and Aging. Endocrinology and Metabolism Clinics of North America, pp. 893–917. Saunders, Philadelphia 1987.

[39] Strollo, F., J. Harlin, H. Hernandez-Monets et al.: Qualitative and quantitative differences in the isoelectrofocusing profile of biologically active lutropin in the blood of normally menstruating and post-menopausal women. Acta. Endocrinol. 97 (1981) 166–175.

[40] Timiras, P. S.: Neuroendocrinology of aging. In: J. Meites (ed.): Neuroendocrinology of Aging, pp. 5–29. Plenum Press, New York 1983.

[41] Tsai, C. C., S. S. C. Yen: Acute effects of intravenous infusion of 17β-estradiol on gonadotropin release in pre- and post-menopausal women. J. Clin. Endocrinol. Metab. 32 (1971) 766–769.

[42] Weiland, N. G., P. M. Wise: Aging progressively decreases the densities and alters the diurnal rhythms of a1-adrenergic receptors in selected hypothalamic regions. Endocrinology 126 (1990) 2392–2397.

[43] Wide, L., B. M. Hobson: Qualitative difference in follicle-stimulating hormone activity in the pituitary of young women compared to that of men and elderly women. J. Clin. Endocrinol. Metab. 56 (1983) 371–375.

[44] Wise, P. M.: The role of the hypothalamus in aging of the female reproductive system. J. Steroid Biochem. 27 (1987) 713–719.

[45] Witkins, J. W.: Morphology of luteinizing hormone-releasing hormone neurons as a function of age and hormonal condition in the male rat. Neuroendocrinology 49 (1989) 344–348.

[46] Yen, S. C. C., C. C. Tsai, F. Naftolin et al.: Pulsatile patterns of gonadotropin release in subjects with and without ovarian function. J. Clin. Endocrinol. Metab. 24 (1972) 671–675.

[47] Yen, S. S. C.: The biology of the menopause. J. Reprod. Med. 18 (1977) 287–296.

[48] Yen, S. S. C.: The hypothalamic control of pituitary hormone secretion. In: S. S. C. Yen, R. B. Jaffe (eds.): Reproductive Endocrinology, pp. 65–104. Saunders, Philadelphia 1991.

Estrogen-progestagen substitution during late postmenopause and old-age

C. Lauritzen

The problems

The female gonads, in contrast to testes, cease to function during the sixth decade of life. As the age expectancy is about 80 years for women, they have to live the last third of their lives without the beneficial effects of their ovarian hormones. Certainly oophoropause and menopause are not diseases. However, some symptoms of estrogen deficiency may be so distressing that the individual will feel ill and really disabled, especially as concerns nervousness, sleep disturbances and depressive mood. However, the late consequences of estrogen deficiency such as osteoporosis and cardiovascular diseases are certainly grave diseases.

The demographic argument

As the proportion of the aged population increases, the problem of treatment, but even more so, that of prevention of disease accompanying old-age, becomes increasingly important.

Main causes of morbidity and mortality in women

The main causes of morbidity and mortality in women are indeed cardiovascular diseases, followed by osteoporosis. The number of deaths due to myocardial infarction are six times greater than those caused by mammary, uterine or ovarian cancer combined. The number of deaths caused by osteoporosis is two times greater than the number caused by all gynecological cancers.

Prevention rather than treatment

The fact that a long-term postmenopausal estrogen substitution is capable of favorably influencing arteriosclerosis and its sequelae such as myocardial infarction and cerebrovascular bleeding as well as osteoporosis and bone fractures, provides a strong argument for prevention of these diseases by giving ovarian hormones.

It is a fact that estrogens are not only sexual hormones, but much more growth factors and metabolically active hormones. They stimulate cell division, growth, blood perfusion of sexual organs, of the skin and of many other organs of the body. Estrogens exert a positive influence on lipoproteins and bone mineral content. They improve fitness, well-being and secure life quality.

Psyche

As concerns psychic conditions, estrogens improve concentration attention, memory, psychomotoric skill and the ability to learn and establish social contacts. Depressive mood is also favorably influenced.

Urogenital symptoms

Postmenopausal women have an increased incidence of urogenital infections. Estrogen substitution prevents senile colpitis, cyto-urethritis, urge-incontinence, vaginal decensus and stress incontinence to some degree.

Skin

How old a person really is, is evidenced by the condition of their skin. Estrogens stimulate epidermal proliferation, blood perfusion, water-binding capacity and elasticity by stimulation of hyaluronic acid and connective tissue collagen. Also, the state of the mucosa is improved by estrogens.

Prevention of osteoporosis

Osteoporosis is a disease predominantly found in postmenopausal women. In that age there is a high prevalence of fractures of the vertebral spine, forearm and hip. Invalidity and chronic pain are frequent consequences. The post-fracture mortality is up to 15%. The costs for treatment of these sequelae are high. Long-term estrogen substitution will prevent 60−95% of the bone fractures.

Prevention of cardiovascular and cerebrovascular diseases

As concerns cardiovascular diseases, long-term estrogen substitution will prevent about 50% of the myocardial infarctions and cerebrovascular bleedings, and about 50% of the deaths due to these causes. The preventive effect of estrogen substitution will prevent about 600 deaths per 100,000 women of the climacteric age group per year. The preventive effect is even maintained for some years after withdrawal of the hormones.

Begin and duration of estrogen-progestagen substitution

When should the treatment begin and how long should treatment be? It would be optimal so start substitution shortly before or at menopause. The substitution should be maintained as long as long as possible up to old age, in extreme cases to the end of life. To secure a sufficient effect on cardiovascular diseases and osteoporosis, a 10-year substitution would be desirable.

Patient fears

Many patients feel anxious about presumed severe side-effects of estrogens such as thromboembolism and gynecological cancer. However, in contrast to the contraceptive pill, natural estrogens and progestagens given in substitution doses do not increase the risk for thromboembolic diseases. While an estrogen only monotherapy will increase the risk for endometrial cancer, addition of a progestagen reduces endometrial cancer risk for 80% as compared to untreated controls. Ovarian cancer risk is reduced by estrogen + progestagen for about 50%, mammary cancer risk for 20%.

Contraindications

There are only a few contraindications for an estrogen substitution, namely mammary cancer and perhaps some cases of endometrial cancer. Exceptions are, however, possible. In mammary cancer cases which are receptor negative, an estrogen-progestagen substitution can be given. Endometrial cancer, properly treated and probably cured, is no longer a contraindication. In ovarian cancer, a posttreatment substitution will improve the prognosis.

Hypertension, varicosis, myocardial infarction, thromboembolism, cerebral bleeding in the patient's history, diabetes, otosclerosis and malign melanoma are no longer contraindications for a substitution.

Side-effects

Side-effects are rare and result for the most part from too high dosages. Reduction of estrogen-progestagen dose will abolish the symptoms. In risk cases small doses of hormones can be given and transdermal application is preferable. The disadvantages of withholding an estrogen substitution always have to be weighted against the virtual risk of substitution; which can be minimized by properly individualized dosing, mode of application and the addition of a progestagen.

Modes of application

Oral, transdermal (patches and gels) as well as injections, vaginal rings, subcutaneous plants and rectal or vaginal applications are possible and guarantee a broad spectrum of individualization.

A progestagen is usually added to exclude undesired symptoms of a one-sided estrogen-effect. In cases of hysterectomy, a progestagen medication is not necessary. If progestagens are not well tolerated it is possible to give a progestagen for 12 days every 3−6 months only to cause secretory change of the endometrium and withdrawal bleeding.

Conclusion

In conclusion, long-term estrogen-progestagen substitution in female menopause, postmenopause and old-age has a high-preventive effect in avoiding unnecessary complaints and diseases in older women. It would be desirable to warrant the beneficial effects of a long-term estrogen-progestagen substitution to more women than receive it.

Age-dependent changes in growth hormone secretion in adults

J. D. Veldhuis, A. Iranmanesh

Abstract

Profound changes in growth hormone (GH) secretion occur during the course of healthy aging. For example, even prior to puberty pulsatile GH secretion occurs with diurnal rhythmicity, and these patterns are amplified 2−3 fold by mid-puberty as sex steroid hormone concentrations increase. Despite a continuing adult level of estrogen or testosterone, pulsatile GH secretion declines primarily in amplitude in young postpubertal adulthood (ages 18−25). Thereafter, a further age-related fall in GH secretion occurs in men. Our recent use of deconvolution analysis has disclosed specific mechanisms by which mean serum GH concentrations begin to fall exponentially in the mid-third decade of life. Particularly, by sampling blood at 10-minute intervals for 24 hours in a cohort of men whose ages ranged from 21 to 72 years, and by applying quantitative deconvolution analysis to identify underlying GH secretory bursts and calculate GH half-life simultaneously, we have observed: (1) a significantly negative effect of increasing age on the number of detectable GH secretory bursts in healthy men; (2) a significantly negative correlation between increasing body mass index (a measure of adiposity) or percentage body fat (determined by underwater weighing) and the amplitude of spontaneous GH secretory bursts in healthy men; (3) a small (30%) but significant decline in the calculated half-life of endogenous GH in middle-aged individuals especially those with relative or absolute increases in adiposity; (4) a decline in the mass of GH secreted per event with increasing relative adiposity; (5) evidence of nyctohemeral rhythmicity in plasma GH concentrations but at reduced amplitude, and (6) strongly positive correlations between the serum total or free testosterone concentration and the mean serum GH concentration, daily GH secretion rate, mass of GH secreted per burst, and the GH half-life. In contrast, in this population of healthy aging men, we found no correlation between serum estradiol concentrations and specific measures of GH secretion or metabolic removal.

In summary, mean plasma GH concentrations in healthy men fall exponentially with both increasing body mass index and advancing age, and the interaction between these two variables in reducing GH secretion is highly significant. The serum testosterone concentration is a strongly positive predictor of the mean serum GH concentration, as well as of specific indices of GH secretion (mass of hormone released per burst, and total daily GH production rate) and GH kinetics (GH half-life). Accordingly, we suggest that the profound fall in serum GH concentrations in healthy older men reflects at least the combined 3-fold influences of age, alterations in body composition (increasing relative adiposity), and declining serum testosterone concentrations. The role of other factors such as altered sleep, reduced vigorous exercise, and age-related variations in dietary intake, etc. in attenuating GH secretion in healthy older individuals will require further study.

Introduction

Clinical investigations over the last two decades have uniformly disclosed a significant decline in mean serum GH concentrations in the course of healthy aging in men and women [1, 6, 11, 16, 17, 19−22, 31, 33, 34, 41, 54, 57, 58, 70, 83, 91]. Moreover, specific secretagogues of GH typically have reduced efficacy in elderly individuals, e. g. sleep [6, 54], alpha agonists [21], cholinergic agonists [19], growth-hormone releasing hormone (GHRH) [19, 20, 22, 31, 43, 52, 61], etc. However, the precise mechanisms that underlie the fall in mean plasma GH concentrations and attenuated GH release in response to specific secretagogues in the course of healthy aging in men and women are not known.

We have utilized the novel analytical technique of deconvolution analysis [72, 78] to evaluate the neuroendocrine mechanisms subserving a decline in serum GH concentrations during healthy aging. Deconvolution analysis permits one to search for specific alterations in the frequency, amplitude, duration, or mass of GH secretory bursts and/or the kinetics of GH removal [72, 73, 78], all of which are plausible points of regulation of pulsatile GH release [23−25, 29, 32−34, 46, 47, 68, 73−75, 79−82, 87, 88, 90]. Indeed, a range of physiological variables including steroid hormone concentrations, relative adiposity, nutrition, sleep, exercise, glucocorticoids, thyroid status, puberty, age and infancy can all modify specific facets of pulsatile GH secretion or its metabolic clearance (reviewed [24, 34, 73]). These environmental and endogenous cues presumably converge on one or more of three primary loci of physiological regulation of GH secretion, namely, hypothalamic somatostatin and growth-hormone releasing hormone (GHRH) secretion, and responsiveness of anterior pituitary somatotropes to inhibition and stimulation by somatostatin and GHRH [7, 18, 38, 42, 44, 49, 59, 63, 66, 67, 86].

Alterations in the pulsatile mode of GH secretion are of considerable pathophysiological interest for several cogent reasons. First, the time course of the trophic GH stimulus can significantly influence target tissue responses [4, 8, 12, 35−37, 48, 60, 64]. For example, the induction of gene transcripts for IGF-I in muscle or liver, the expression of hepatic cytochrome P450 enzymes, or prolactin and GH receptors, linear bone growth, and the appearance of IGF-I and/or IGF-binding protein 3 in plasma are all influenced by the mode of delivery of GH; namely, whether the target tissue is exposed to pulses of GH or continuous unvarying concentrations. Secondly, an examination of the pulsatile mode of GH secretion is valuable, because it gives indirect **in vivo** insights into the interaction between hypothalamic releasing and inhibitory factors and the contemporaneous responsiveness of anterior pituitary somatotrope cells [7, 18, 38, 44, 49, 59, 63]. Thirdly, the pulsatile mode of GH secretion is subject to exquisite pathophysiological regulation by sex steroid hormones, glucocorticoids, body composition, puberty, age, infancy, nutrition, sleep, exercise, thyroid hormone status, and hepatic or renal disease (reviewed [24, 34, 73]). Consequently, to gain further understanding of the mechanisms subserving the effects of age on the somatotropic axis is man, we have evaluated in detail specific alterations in the pulsatile mode of GH secretion as a function of age in healthy men over a five decade age span. We have applied the technique of deconvolution analysis to estimate the number, amplitude, duration, and mass of individual GH secretory bursts and simultaneously calculated the apparent half-life of endogenous GH [72, 78].

Technical limitations in evaluating in vivo pulsatile GH secretion and metabolic clearance

Studies of neuroendocrine axes require intensive and extended venous sampling to characterize spontaneous profiles of pulsatile hormone release accurately [13, 23, 69, 88]. Indeed, blood withdrawal at 5 minute intervals for 24 hours provides a significantly higher estimate of the number of GH secretory bursts compared to sampling at 15, 20, or 30 minute intervals [23]. Conventional radioimmunoassays and immunoradiometric assays predominantly measure total GH in plasma, rather than just the putatively biologically active free GH [79]. Moreover, most assays do not have adequate low-end sensitivity to measure serum GH concentrations in all samples obtained during the awake fed state, when serum GH concentrations often fall below 0.1 ng/ml [73]. Indeed, as illustrated in Fig. 1, even by middle age there is a profound fall in mean serum GH concentrations so that the majority of daytime samples do not contain detectable GH [33, 74]. In contrast, recently developed chemiluminescence assays have achieved considerably higher sensitivity (in the range of $2-5$ pg/ml), which allows all serum GH concentrations to be measured during the course of a full day and night in healthy, middle aged men, including subjects who are obese or hypothyroid and hence have even lower mean serum GH concentrations (Fig. 1).

IRMA

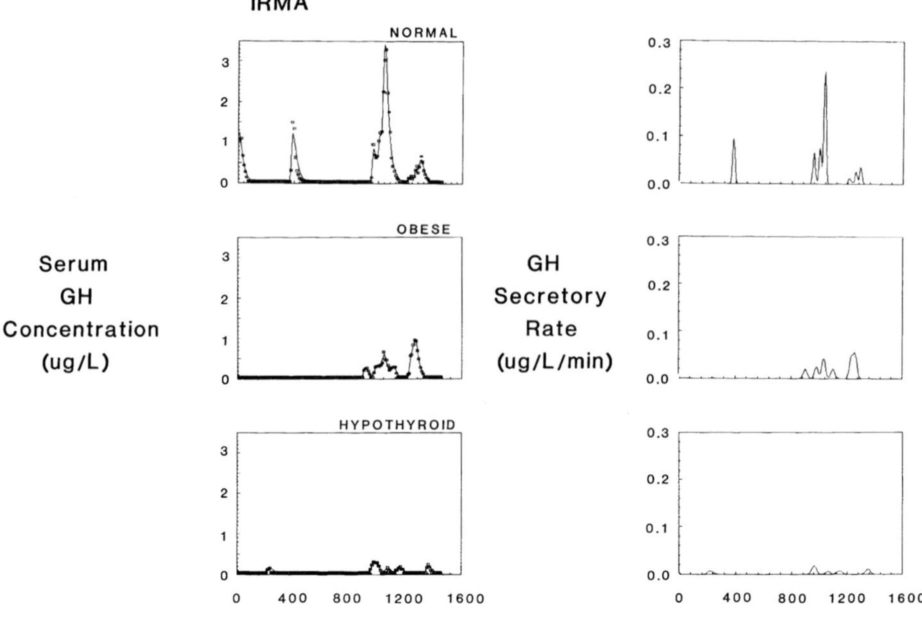

Chemiluminescence

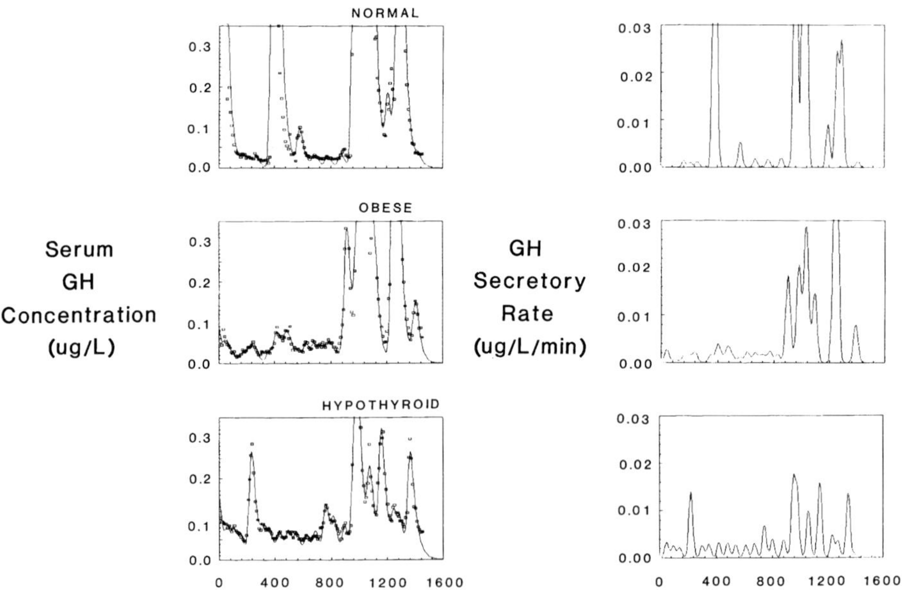

As reviewed elsewhere in greater detail [14, 23, 73, 77], the identification of GH release episodes in plasma is dependent not only upon the frequency of blood sampling and the sensitivity, precision, and reliability of the GH assay, but also on the analytical tool used to identify significant release episodes. For example, the vast majority of studies evaluating episodic GH release have utilized so-called discrete peak detection algorithms. One such technique, Cluster analysis, which is illustrated in the top panel of Fig. 2, is designed to search for significant increases or decreases in serum hormone concentrations [69, 76]. However, different types of discrete algorithms may behave rather discrepantly even when applied to the same data sets, and are subject to the limitation that no cognizance is taken of subject-specific hormone half-life [69, 72, 73, 76, 78]. The latter consideradion is important, because available studies of the metabolic clearance rate of GH have revealed up to 4-fold variability within healthy apparently homogeneous populations of study subjects [2, 3, 10, 15, 26, 27, 30, 41, 45, 50, 51, 56, 64, 65]. Thus, intersubject variation in GH half-life may contribute significantly to differences in serum GH concentrations. Accordingly, analytically more penetrating techniques such as deconvolution analysis are helpful in evaluating the frequency, amplitude, duration and mass of underlying GH secretory episodes, when such techniques are able to adjust for the expected effects of predicted or calculated GH half-lives on the serum GH concentration profile [72, 78]. As discussed below, deconvolution methods may either depend upon **a priori** determinations of GH half-life, or estimate the apparent GH half-life in each individual subject (multi-parameter deconvolution method).

Deconvolution analysis as a tool to evaluate in vivo GH secretion and metabolic removal

Deconvolution analysis refers to the calculation of hormone secretion given information or assumptions concerning GH metabolic removal rates [14, 72,

Fig. 1 Comparison between the immunoradiometric assay (IRMA) and the chemiluminescent assay for GH in a normal middle-aged subject, an obese individual, and a hypothyroid man. In both assays, the serial serum GH concentrations in blood collected at 10-minute intervals for 24 hours are shown in the left column. The corresponding calculated GH secretion rates (estimated by multi-parameter deconvolution analysis) are given in the right column. Note that for the chemiluminescent assay, the vertical scales have been expanded 10-fold to illustrate the presence of pulsatile GH secretion even at extremely low serum GH concentrations. In the three individuals illustrated here, the number of detectable GH secretory bursts rose from a mean value of 8 estimated in the IRMA to 18 estimated in the same serum samples following chemiluminescence assay. Consequently, most available RIA and IRMA techniques underestimate absolute GH secretory burst frequency to a significant degree. (Unpublished observations.)

73, 77, 78]. In general, two principal classes of deconvolution analysis can be used to study pulsatile hormone secretion **in vivo**: see Fig. 3. First, most earlier and many recent methods require **a priori** knowledge of the hormone half-life in the study population under consideration, and assume that this general estimate of hormone half-life can be applied reasonably among different subjects and at different times. Given knowledge of the hormone half-life, this kind of

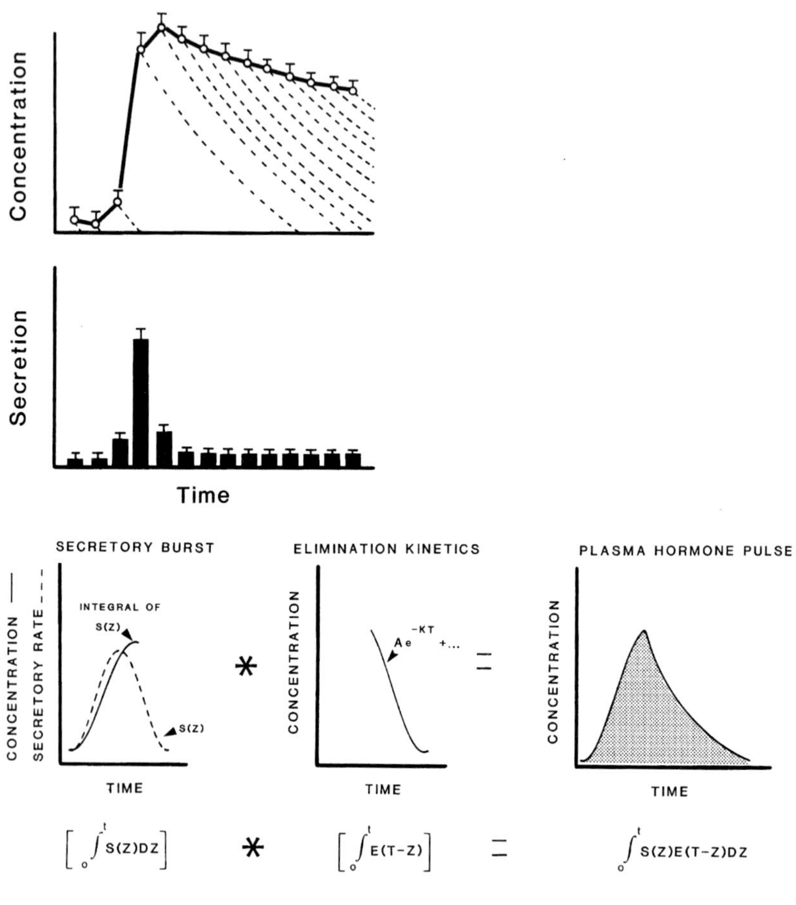

$$\left[\int_{0}^{t} S(Z)DZ \right] \quad * \quad \left[\int_{0}^{t} E(T-Z) \right] \quad = \quad \int_{0}^{t} S(Z)E(T-Z)DZ$$

Fig. 2 Schematic presentations of the concepts underlying our waveform-independent deconvolution algorithm (Panel A, PULSE), and our multi-parameter deconvolution technique (Panel B, DECONV). In PULSE, **a priori** knowledge of the hormone half-life is required typically in the form of biexponential kinetics [78]. Sample-by-sample secretion rates are then calculated based on conservation of mass. In contrast, in DECONV (multi-parameter method), both hormone half-life **and** secretory burst measures (amplitude, number, mass, and duration) are calculated in each subject. Both methodologies reveal an exclusively burst-like mode of GH secretion in normal individuals (see Fig. 3) when RIA or IRMA methods are used, but basal GH secretion also in the chemiluminescence assay.

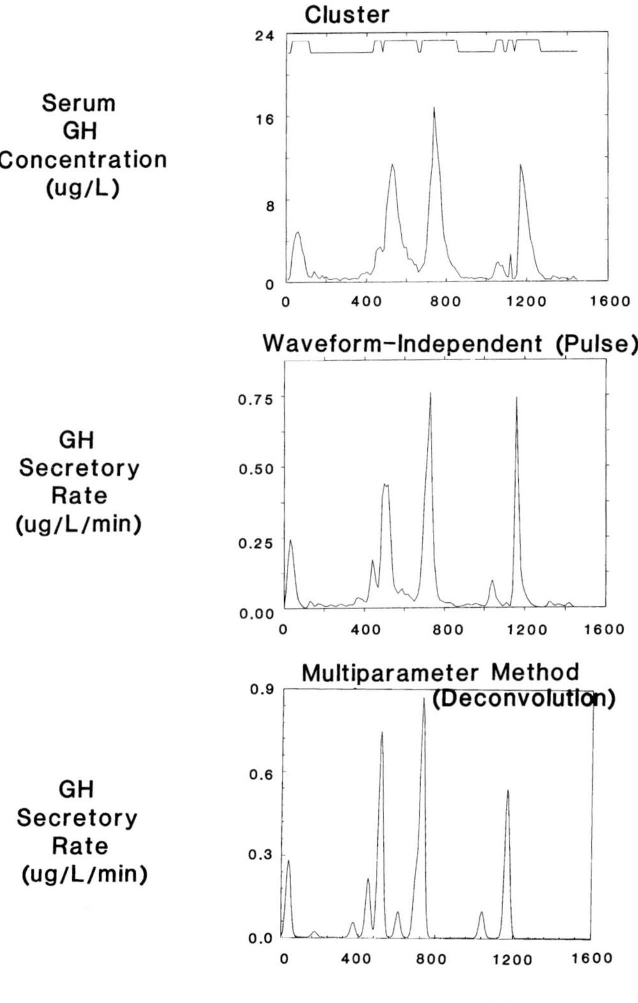

Fig. 3   Comparison of the evaluation of a 24 hour serum GH concentration profile by a discrete pulse detection algorithm (Cluster) [76], by a waveform-independent deconvolution technique (PULSE) [78], and a multi-parameter method (DECONV) [72]. The upper panel gives the serum GH concentrations measured in blood collected at 10-minute intervals for 24 hours in one healthy young man. Above the measured profile, we illustrate the Cluster-identified individual peaks by the schematized reflections above the data. In the middle panel, a waveform-independent deconvolution procedure (PULSE) was employed assuming a two-compartment GH disappearance profile consisting of a 3.5 minute rapid half-life phase, a 21 minute slow half-life phase, and a relative amplitude of the slower component of 63% [15]. The GH secretory profile in the lower panel was derived by multi-parameter deconvolution (DECONV), in which the number, location, duration, and mass of underlying GH secretory bursts and the half-life of endogenous GH are estimated simultaneously [72]. This methodology assumes that either a skewed or a Gaussian waveform can be used to approximate the underlying hormone secretory burst, whereas the waveform-independent (PULSE) methodology (middle panel) calculates GH secretion rates in each sample with no assumption about the presence or absence of pulsatility or basal secretion or any particular waveform (Fig. 2). Of interest, the waveform-independent and the multi-parameter method yield rather similar inferences regarding the underlying nature of pulsatile GH secretion in this healthy young subject.

deconvolution analysis predicts the secretion rates that would be required to achieve the observed serum hormone concentrations in each blood sample [78]. We illustrate our recent formulation of this kind of method, and its application to a serum GH concentration profile in Fig. 2 (middle panel). We call this approach **waveform-independent**, because assumptions about the secretory waveform (e. g. burst and/or tonic secretion) are kept to a minimum, but it has the disadvantage that the hormone half-life must be known or assumed to be uniform in all study subjects. The latter assumption is probably an oversimplification for biological data, since substantial variability typically exists for hormone half-lives measured in different individual healthy subjects (vide supra). Moreover, in pathological conditions, or in selected physiological states, the half-life of hormone removal may be altered, sometimes markedly; e. g. in obesity, the half-life of GH is decreased [74, 85], and in liver and renal disease the half-life of GH is significantly increased [5, 50, 80]. For example, recently we have observed that in seven men with chronic liver disease the calculated half-life of endogenous GH was 43 ± 4.0 minutes, which compares with a control value of 24 ± 3.6 minutes and a post liver-transplantation value of 21 ± 3.4 minutes (Cuneo and Veldhuis, unpublished observations). Accordingly, we believe that deconvolution analysis wherever possible should be capable of identifying shortened or prolonged half-lives of GH anticipated in the various clinical contexts.

A second model of deconvolution analysis has been referred to as the **multiparameter technique**, since estimates are made of **both** hormone secretion **and** removal rates [14, 72, 73, 77, 78]: see Fig. 3. For example, if a presumptive waveform for underlying hormone secretory bursts is assumed (e. g. either skewed or symmetric secretory bursts of individually varying amplitude), then multi-parameter deconvolution analysis allows one to estimate the number, duration, amplitude, and mass of significant underlying secretory bursts **as well as** simultaneously estimate the half-life of endogenous hormone removal [72, 78]. Application of this technique to a serum GH concentration profile is illustrated in Fig. 2 (bottom panel). Multi-parameter deconvolution has revealed a wide range of GH secretory burst amplitude, mass, and duration, and in some cases modulation of GH secretory pulse frequency as well as the rate of GH metabolic removal (reviewed [24, 34, 73]). Some of these physiological and pathological regulators of GH secretion or metabolic clearance are summarized briefly below.

Pathophysiological regulation of pulsatile GH secretion and clearance

Steroid hormones are dominant stimulators of pulsatile GH secretion, as inferred indirectly from studies of healthy puberty as well as more directly by the administration of estrogen or testosterone to children with delayed pubertal onset [46, 47, 68]. In general, the administration of estrogen or an aromatizable androgen such as testosterone increases the amplitude (and mass per burst) of pulsatile GH release without altering the apparent half-life of GH removal [47, 68]. A very small amount of sex steroid hormone (e. g. 100 ng/kg ethinyl estradiol orally for 1 week) can increase the amplitude of deconvolution-estimated GH secretory bursts, which results in an increased mass of GH secreted per pulse [68]: Fig. 4. A similar effect can be achieved with testosterone [47], and in a small study was observed in five children treated with the nonaromatizable androgen, oxandrolone [47]. Moreover, during normal puberty, there is an approximate doubling of GH secretory burst amplitude and mass, with no change

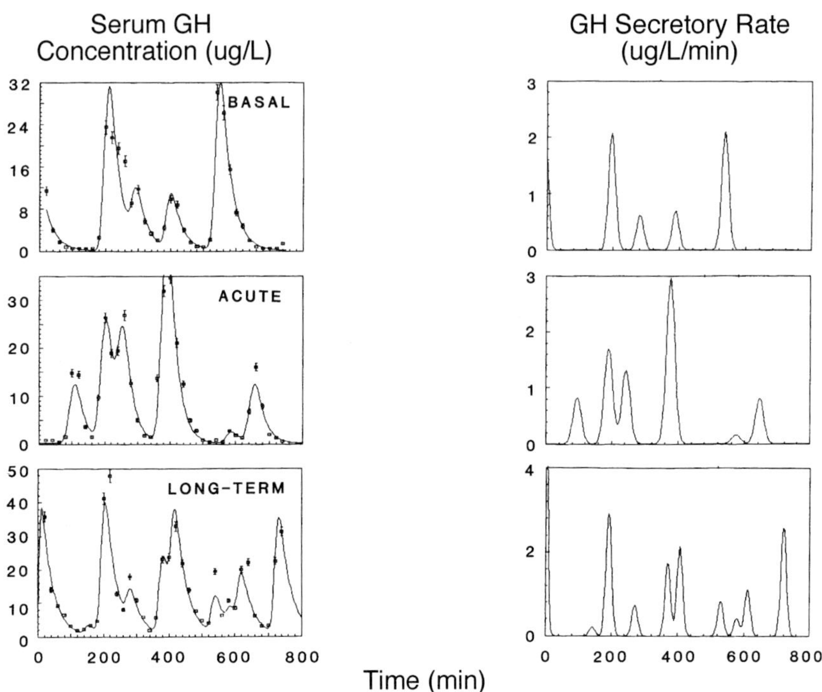

Fig. 4 Stimulatory effects of acute or longer-term estrogen administration on pulsatile GH secretion in a young prepubertal girl with Turner's syndrome. The left panels denote the overnight profiles of serum GH concentrations assayed in blood sampled at 20 minute intervals basally (prior to estrogen administration), acutely (after 1 week of estrogen, 100 ng/kg ethinyl estradiol orally daily), and longer term (4−6 weeks). The corresponding right-hand panels depict the multi-parameter deconvolution estimates of pulsatile GH secretion in the same subject. Note the prominent effect of estrogen on the amplitude of GH secretory bursts. Similar effects occur in response to testosterone administration in boys with constitutionally delayed puberty [47]. Data are adapted with permission from Mauras, N., J. D. Veldhuis: Increased hGH production rate after low-dose estrogen therapy in prepubertal girls with Turner's syndrome. Pediatric. Res. 28(6) (1990) 626−630.

in the frequency of pulsatile GH release or its apparent half-life [46]: Fig. 5. This illustrates the 24 hour profiles of pulsatile serum GH concentrations in early and late puberty and in young adulthood. We present the 24-hour fitted profiles (predicted by the deconvolution analysis) as well as the estimated underlying GH secretory bursts. Of note, there is a marked increase in GH secretory burst amplitude in late puberty. This increase disappears in adulthood, when GH secretion returns to values similar to those of prepuberty.

Another prominent regulator of GH secretion is nutrition and relative adiposity [25, 28, 33, 57, 74]. For example, short-term fasting increases both the amplitude and detectable frequency of pulsatile GH secretion in healthy young men [25]. Conversely, relative or absolute obesity is accompanied by significant suppression of the amplitude of pulsatile GH secretion, as well as a lesser fall in GH half-life (resulting in more rapid metabolic removal of GH) [33, 74]. The precise metabolic or endocrine or other signals that promote increased GH secretion in response to nutrient restriction, and conversely those that suppress GH secretion in over-feeding or obesity, have not been identified. Available clinical studies indicate that GH release in response to L-dopa, insulin, exercise,

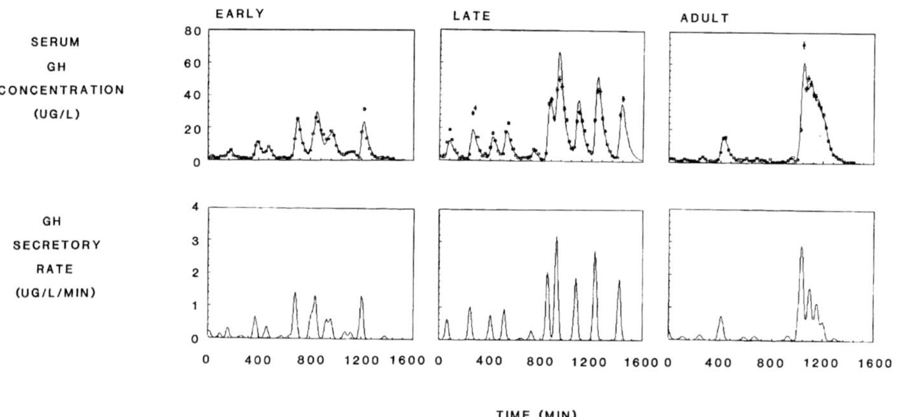

Fig. 5 Serum GH concentration profiles in early and late pubertal boys compared to an adult male. The three upper profiles show serum immunoreactive GH concentrations measured in blood samples collected in 20-minute intervals for 24 hours in the three individual subjects. The continuous curves through the measured serum GH concentrations are predicted by multi-parameter deconvolution analysis [72, 78]. The three lower panels depict the calculated GH secretory rates, which conform to punctuated episodes of GH secretion. Note the two-fold increase in GH secretory burst amplitude in late puberty and return to prepubertal secretory burst amplitudes in adulthood. Data are adapted with permission from Martha Jr., P. M., K. M. Goorman, R. M. Blizzard, A. D. Rogol, J. D. Veldhuis: Endogenous growth hormone secretion and clearance rates in normal boys as determined by deconvolution analysis: relationship of age, pubertal status and body mass. J. Clin. Endocrinol. Metab. 74 (1992) 336–344.

sleep, and GHRH is reduced [39, 40, 53, 62, 84, 89]. Single doses of cholinergic agonists only partially restore GH secretion in obesity [9], whereas weight loss is effective in enhancing GH production [89]. The basis for accelerated metabolic clearance (reduced GH half-life) in obesity is not known, but has been inferred in both the human by deconvolution analysis [74] and the orchidectomized rhesus monkey by steady-state infusions of recombinant human GH [10]. Consequently, hyposomatotropism associated with obesity can be accounted for by at least dual mechanisms: (1) suppression of the pulse amplitude (and mass) of GH secretory bursts [33, 74]; and (2) increased metabolic clearance of GH (or an increased GH distribution volume) [10, 74]. In relation to the attenuation of GH secretory burst amplitude, either increased hypothalamic somatostatin inhibitory tone, or decreased hyopthalamic GHRH release, and/or altered pituitary responsiveness to these regulating peptides may be responsible.

Sleep also represents a potent regulator of pulsatile GH secretion. Recent studies using 30-second blood sampling [29] or less frequent blood sampling combined with the injection of GHRH at various stages of sleep [67] imply that stages III and IV of slow-wave sleep coincide with the majority of GH secretory bursts over the nighttime, and that somatostatin withdrawal (with or without enhanced endogenous GHRH secretion) is important in augmenting GH secretion at this time.

Exercise also represents a potent immediate stimulus to GH secretion (reviewed [34]). In addition, our recent studies indicate that long-term endurance training promotes an approximate two-fold increase in mean (24-hour) serum GH concentrations in healthy young women [87]. This increase is due to a doubling of GH pulse amplitude [87]. Deconvolution analysis and/or direct measurements of GH secretion and clearance will be required to determine whether the increase in serum GH pulse amplitude following long-term physical training is due to an increased mass of GH secreted per burst, a prolongation of the secretory burst duration, the appearance of basal GH secretion (if any), and/or a decline in the rate of GH removal from blood.

The above primary regulators of pulsatile GH secretion are of particular interest in this overview on aging, because each is or may be altered to some degree in the course of normal aging: see below.

Multifactorial influence of age on pulsatile GH secretion in the human

As shown in Fig. 6, healthy men exhibit a pronounced decline in pulsatile GH secretion with significant suppression of the frequency of detectable GH secretory bursts during normal aging [33, 74]. As noted above, because of the inability to detect serum GH concentrations below approximately 0.1 ng/ml in conventional immunoradiometric and radioimmunoassays, the **absolute** frequency of pulsatile GH secretion cannot be estimated accurately [14, 33, 73, 77, 78]. Indeed, it is theoretically possible that aging is associated with a suppression of GH secretory burst amplitude alone, resulting in very attenuated GH secretory bursts that are no longer detectable (see Fig. 1, and earlier comments). This would result in an **apparent** decrease in GH secretory burst frequency. Of interest, there is still a diurnal rhythmicity of GH release in older individuals, since decreases occur in both daytime and nighttime GH concentrations [33, 74].

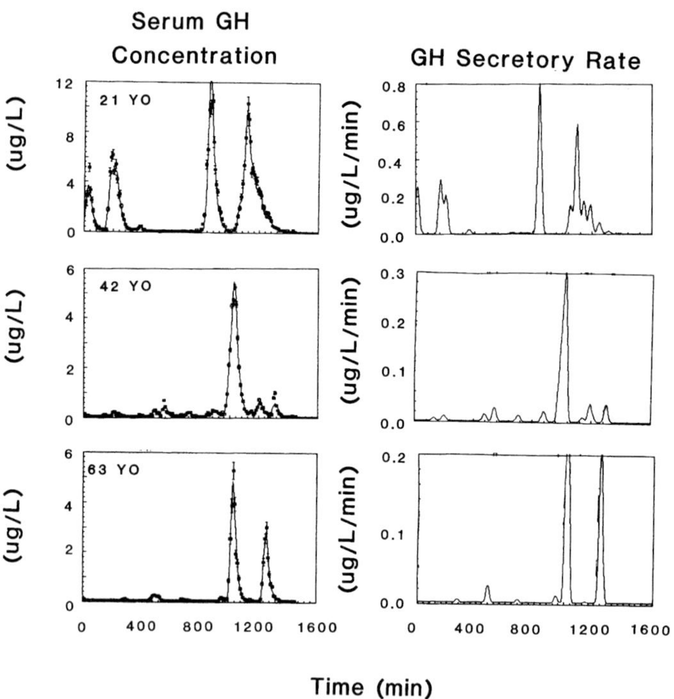

Fig. 6a   Influence of age on 24-hour serum GH concentration profiles and pulsatile GH secretion in healthy men. The left column of panels gives the 24-hour serum GH concentration profiles in three men who underwent blood sampling at 10-minute intervals for 24 hours. Profiles are illustrated for men aged 21 (upper), 42 (middle), and 63 (lower). The right column of plots depicts the multi-parameter deconvolution estimates of GH secretion over time. Note the differences in scales across the three age groups to accommodate the marked changes in GH secretory rates that occur with healthy aging. There is a decline in the detectable GH secretory burst frequency with aging, which may relate to either a true fall in GH secretory burst frequency or reflect the limitation of current immunoradiometric assays with sensitivities of approximately 0.1 ng/ml (see Fig. 1).

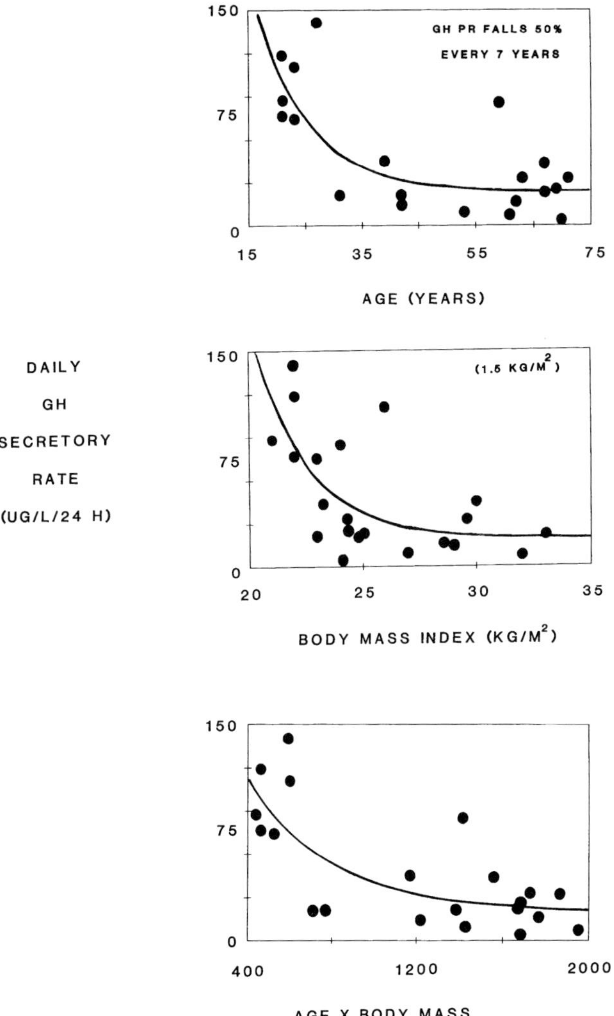

Fig. 6b   Individual and combined negative influences of age (left), body mass index (BMI, middle), and the combined effects of age and BMI (right) on daily GH secretion rates in a cohort of 21 healthy men. Data are adapted with permission from Iranmanesh, A., G. Lizarralde, J. D. Veldhuis: Age and relative adiposity are specific negative determinants of the frequency and amplitude of GH secretory bursts and the half-life of endogenous GH in healthy men. J. Clin. Endocrinol. Metab. 73 (1991) 1081–1088.

Simple linear regression analysis was used initially to assess the relationships between age and specific measures of GH secretion or half-life. Fig. 7 illustrates the negative correlation of age with GH half-life (r = −0.61, P = 0.003), and the inverse relationship between age and GH secretory burst frequency (number of detectable GH secretory events/24 hours, r = −0.77, P = 0.001).

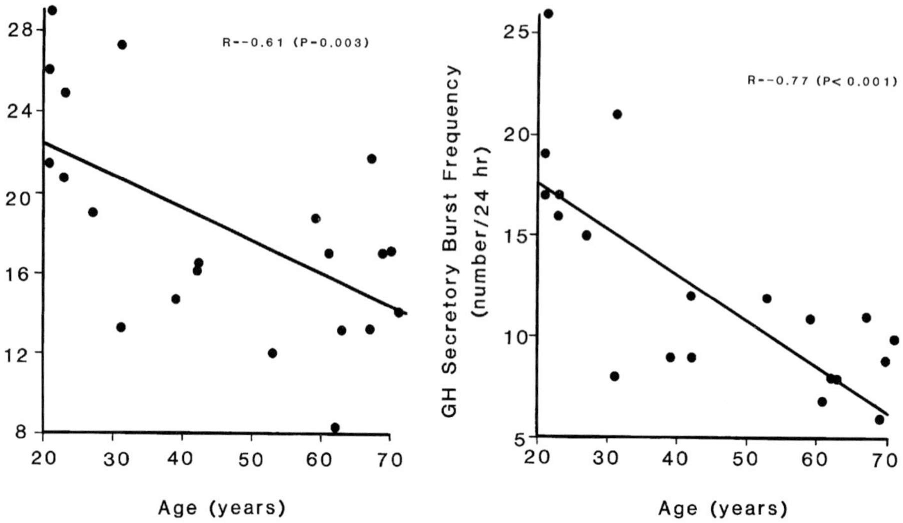

Fig. 7 Negative correlations between age and calculated GH half-life, as well as between age and detectable GH secretory burst frequency in 21 healthy men. Twenty-one men underwent blood sampling at 10-minute intervals for 24 hours, and the subsequent immunoradiometric GH profiles were subjected to multi-parameter deconvolution analysis (Fig. 2). This latter technique permitted us to estimate detectable GH secretory burst frequency, as well as endogenous GH half-life. The r values denote the correlation coefficients for simple linear regression of age on GH half-life and GH secretory burst frequency. Data are adapted with permission from Iranmanesh, A., G. Lizarralde, J. D. Veldhuis: Age and relative adiposity are specific negative determinants of the frequency and amplitude of GH secretory bursts and the half-life of endogenous GH in healthy men. J. Clin. Endocrinol. Metab. 73 (1991) 1981–1088.

Multiple linear regression analysis in our cohort of more than 20 healthy men spanning 5 decades in age revealed that age was a strongly negative determinant of detectable GH secretory burst frequency (P = 0.0005), whereas body mass index (a measure of relative adiposity) was not [33, 74]. The combination of age and body mass index negatively influenced GH secretory burst frequency (detectable events/24 hours) with a R-squared value of 0.64 (r = −0.80, P = 0.0003). The effect of age on detectable GH secretory event frequency was specific, since age did not affect the GH secretory burst duration or mass. GH secretory burst amplitude was negatively specified jointly by age and body mass index (r = −0.61, P = 0.026), but this effect was largely attributed to body mass index only (P = 0.031). Moreover, GH half-life was negatively correlated with age (P = 0.024) and body mass index (P = 0.045) individually and with age and body mass index considered together (r = −0.70, P = 0.0048). Age and body mass index were individually, and jointly, negative determinants of the plasma IGF-I concentration in these men [33].

From the preceding multiple linear regression analysis of the effects of age and/ or body mass index on specific measures of GH secretion and GH half-life, we can infer that age is the dominant negative determinant of detectable GH secretory burst frequency and the daily GH secretion rate [74]. Body mass index is the dominant negative correlate of GH secretory burst amplitude and mass. The **combined** effects of age and body mass index are prominent negative correlates of apparent GH secretory burst frequency, amplitude, mass per burst, the daily GH secretion rate, and to a lesser extent GH half-life [33, 74]. Both age and body mass index are inversely related to plasma IGF-I concentrations, when age and body mass are considered alone or jointly.

We found by multiple linear regression analysis that body mass index per se (independently of age) is also a negative statistical determinant of daily GH secretion rates [33, 74]. Moreover, as Fig. 8 illustrates in eight individual men (age range 60−72) subjected to underwater weighing to calculate their percentage body fat, we found that percentage body fat is a significant negative correlate of GH secretory burst amplitude (r = −0.713, P = 0.05). Thus, this measure of body composition in some manner covaries negatively with GH secretory rates. Our data do not clarify whether this is a causal connection, or define the direction of causation.

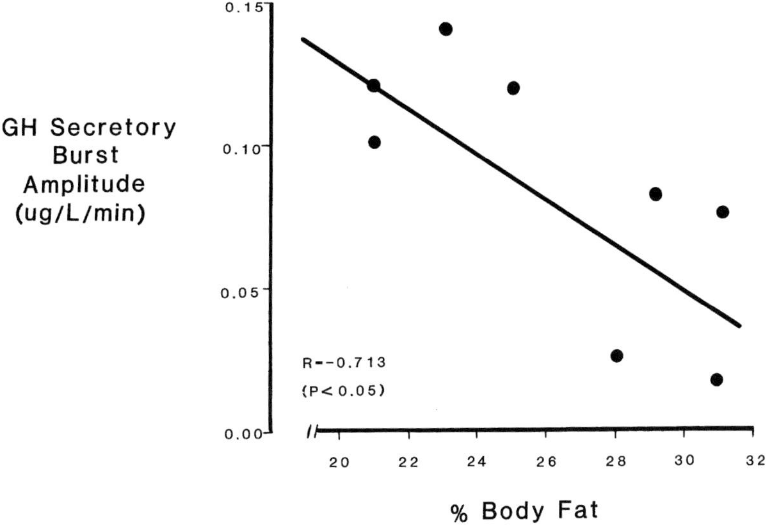

Fig. 8 Negative correlation between the percentage of body fat (determined by underwater weighing) and deconvolution estimates of GH secretory burst amplitude in eight healthy older men. The r value denotes the correlation co-efficient of simple linear regression. Data are adapted with permission from Iranmanesh, A., G. Lizarralde, J. D. Veldhuis: Age and relative adiposity are specific negative determinants of the frequency and amplitude of GH secretory bursts and the half-life of endogenous GH in healthy men. J. Clin. Endocrinol. Metab. 73 (1991) 1081−1088.

Of considerable interest, mean serum GH concentrations in healthy men over a 5-decade age span were strongly positively correlated with serum total (or free) testosterone concentrations (r = +0.717, P < 0.001). In addition, the serum total testosterone concentration was a strongly positive predictor of the GH secretion rate (r = +0.708, P < 0.001), the mass of GH secreted per burst (r = +0.508, P = 0.022), and the GH half-life (r = +0.595, P = 0.006): see Fig. 9. These findings in a group of healthy men suggest that falling androgens contribute to the age-related decline in GH concentrations [33, 74]. Alternatively, serum total and free testosterone concentrations may decline progressively with increasing age, because GH concentrations fall, in view of the putatively trophic role of GH in gonadal physiology [71].

Our analysis of the relationship between plasma IGF-I concentrations and GH dynamics in healthy men indicated that the daily GH secretion rate was strongly positively correlated with the plasma IGF-I concentration (r = +0.584, P < 0.01), as was the GH half-life (r = +0.733, P < 0.005), and GH secretory burst frequency (r = +0.712, P < 0.01). In contrast, GH secretory burst amplitude was not related to plasma IGF-I concentrations in these individuals.

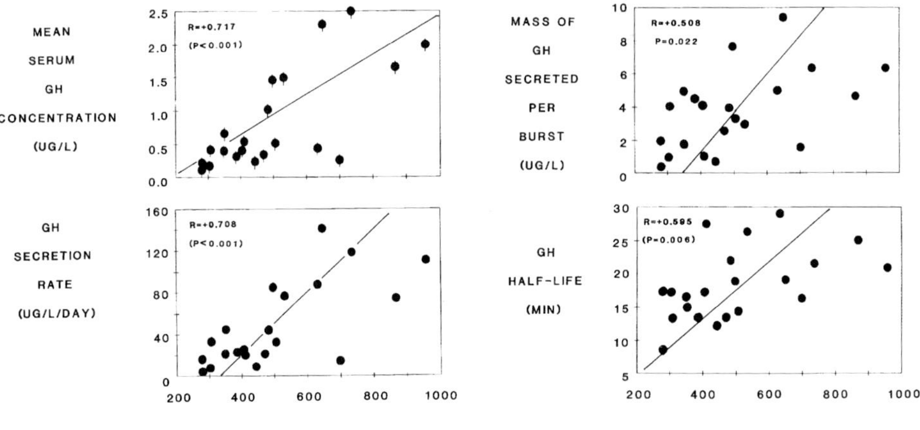

Fig. 9   Linear regression analyses of the relationships between serum total testosterone concentration and: (a) mean serum GH concentration; (b) daily GH secretion rate (micrograms of GH secreted per liter of distribution volume per day); (c) mass of GH secreted per burst (micrograms of GH secreted per liter of distribution volume); and (d) GH half-life (minutes). Data were obtained by multi-parameter deconvolution analysis of 24-hour serum GH profiles collected from 21 healthy men whose ages span 5 decades. Data are adapted with permission from Iranmanesh, A., G. Lizarralde, J. D. Veldhuis: Age and relative adiposity are specific negative determinants of the frequency and amplitude of GH secretory bursts and the half-life of endogenous GH in healthy men. J. Clin. Endocrinol. Metab. 73 (1991) 1081–1088.

Since patterns of sleep can be disrupted in aging individuals (e. g. including a loss of total time in stages III and IV (delta or slow-wave) sleep that are associated with GH secretion) some of the decline in GH production with age might be attributed to processes that result in sleep disruption. In addition, changes in nutritional and exercise-related variables with age may also contribute in part to declining GH secretion. Indeed, other factors such as alterations in the binding affinity of plasma GH binding protein (although total GH binding protein concentrations do not vary greatly with age), the peripheral clearance of GH, and/or increases in the distribution space for GH have not been excluded as potential additional contributors to age-related attenuation of GH secretion.

Summary

Extensive clinical observations over the last two decades indicate that mean serum concentrations of GH decrease with healthy aging in both men and women, and that there are concomitant decreases in secretagogue-stimulated (acute) GH secretion. Further studies suggest that this decline can be partially but not completely opposed by GHRH or cholinergic agonist treatment [19, 31], suggesting a role for GHRH deficiency or somatostatin excess in this process. In addition, the combined administration of arginine and GHRH elicits relatively similar amounts of GH secretion over a broad age range in healthy men [20]. Such findings suggest that the pituitary somatotrope is not irreversibly impaired during healthy aging, and that hypothalamic factors contribute primarily to the hyposomatotropism. Further studies with longer-term cholinergic agonist administration and/or treatment with GHRH or other growth-hormone secretagogues will be required to define the precise mechanisms that result in, and the reversibility of the, suppression of spontaneous GH secretion in older individuals.

Our neuroendocrine studies support the view that both declining serum testosterone concentrations as well as increasing relative adiposity with age are significant co-variates that contribute individually and jointly to age-dependent decreases in GH production. The interaction among decreasing serum testosterone concentrations, increasing adiposity, and increasing age can suppress GH secretion profoundly resulting in GH secretion rates that in the later decades of life are approximately 2−10% those of young adult values. However, other factors are also quite likely in our view, because a significant fall in mean serum GH concentrations as well as GH secretion rates begins exponentially after the second decade of life. For example, in addition to the independent and interactive effects of age, declining sex-steroid hormone concentrations, and increasing relative adiposity on the hyposomatotropism of aging, we believe that changes in central nervous system processes that direct sleep, decreases in strenuous exercise training, and possibly smaller alterations in nutrition may contribute further to reduced GH concentrations in the elderly. Finally, in view of the evident anabolic effects of GH administration in older individuals [55, 57, 58], considerable further clinical investigation is warranted into the pathophysiology of the hyposomatotropism of aging and into pharmacological and non-pharmacological (nutrition, exercise, sleep enhancement) methods of supporting increased GH secretion. As a corollary, further knowledge is needed of the long-term metabolic consequences and other sequelae of restoring serum GH concentrations in the elderly to young adult levels.

Acknowledgements

We thank Patsy Craig for her skillful preparation of the manuscript; Paula P. Azimi for the artwork; Brenda Grisso and Ginger Bauler for performing many of the assays; and Sandra Jackson and the expert nursing staff at the University of Virginia General Clinical Research Center for conduct of the research protocols. This work was supported in part by NIH grant RR-00847 to the General Clinical Research Center of the University of Virginia, Research Career Development Award 1-KO4-HD-00634 (to JDV), NIH-supported Clinfo Data Reduction Systems, Veterans Affairs Merit Review Medical Research Funds (to AI), the Baxter Healthcare Corporation, Round Lake, Illinois (JDV), the University of Virginia Pratt Foundation and Education Enhancement Funds (JDV), and the National Science Foundation Center for Biological Timing (JDV).

References

[1] Bando, H., C. Zhang, Y. Takada et al.: Impaired secretion of growth hormone-releasing hormone, growth hormone, and IGF-I in elderly men. Acta Endocrinol **124** (1991) 31−36.

[2] Baumann, G., M. W. Stolar, T. A. Buchanan: The metabolic clearance, distribution, and degradation of dimeric and monomeric growth hormone (GH): implications for the pattern of circulating GH forms. Endocrinology **119** (1986) 1497.

[3] Baumann, G., M. W. Stolar, T. A. Buchanan: The effect of circulating growth hormone binding protein on metabolic clearance, distribution and degradation of human growth hormone. J. Clin. Endocrinol. Metab. **64** (1987) 657−660.

[4] Bick, T., Z. Hochberg, T. Amit et al.: Roles of pulsatility and continuity of growth hormone (GH) administration in the regulation of hepatic GH-receptors, and circulating GH-binding protein and insulin-like growth factor-I. Endocrinology **131** (1992) 423−429.

[5] Cameron, D. P., H. G. Burger, K. J. Catt et al.: Metabolic clearance of human growth hormone in patients with hepatic and renal failure and in the isolated perifused pig liver. Metabolism **21** (1972) 895−904.

[6] Carlson, H. E., J. C. Gillin, P. Gorden et al.: Absence of sleep related growth hormone peaks in aged normal subjects and in acromegaly. J. Clin. Endocrinol. Metab. 34 (1972) 1102−1105.

[7] Clark, R. G., L. M. S. Carlsson, B. Rafferty et al.: The rebound release of growth hormone (GH) following somatostatin infusion in rats involves hypothalamic GH-releasing factor release. J. Endocrinol. 119 (1988) 397−404.

[8] Clark, R. J., J. O. Jansson, O. G. P. Isaksson et al.: Intravenous growth hormone: growth responses to patterned infusions in hypophysectomized rats. J. Endocrinol. 104 (1985) 53−61.

[9] Cordido, F., F. F. Casanueva, C. Dieguez: Cholinergic receptor activation by pyridostigmine restores growth hormone (GH) responsiveness to GH-releasing hormone administration in obese subjects: evidence for hypothalamic somatostatinergic participation in the blunted GH release of obesity. J. Clin. Endocrinol. Metab. 68 (1989) 290−293.

[10] Dubdey, A. K., A. Ahanukoglu, B. C. Hansen et al.: Metabolic clearance rates of synthetic human growth hormone in lean and obese male rhesus monkeys. J. Clin. Endocrinol. Metab. 67 (1988) 1064−1067.

[11] Dudl, R. J., J. W. Ensinck, H. E. Palmer et al.: Effect of age on growth hormone secretion in man. J. Clin. Endocrinol. Metab. 37 (1973) 11−16.

[12] Eden, S.: Age and sex related differences in episodic growth hormone secretion in the rat. Endocrinology 105 (1979) 555−560.

[13] Evans, W. S., A. C. S. A. Faria, E. Christiansen et al.: Impact of intensive venous sampling on characterization of pulsatile GH release. Am. J. Physiol. 252 (1987) E549−E556.

[14] Faria, A. C. S., L. W. Bekenstein, R. A. Booth Jr. et al.: Pulsatile growth hormone release in normal women during the menstrual cycle. Clin. Endocrinol. 36 (1992) 591−596.

[15] Faria, A. C. S., J. D. Veldhuis, M. O. Thorner et al.: Half-time of endogenous growth hormone (GH) disappearance in normal man after stimulation of GH secretion by GH-releasing hormone and suppression with somatostatin. J. Clin. Endocrinol. Metab. 68 (1989) 535−541.

[16] Finkelstein, J. W., H. P. Roffwarf, R. M. Boyar et al.: Age-related change in the 24-hour spontaneous secretion of growth hormone. J. Clin. Endocrinol. Metab. 36 (1972) 665−670.

[17] Florini, J. R., P. N. Prinz, M. V. Vitiello et al.: Somatomedin-C levels in healthy young and old men: relationship to peak and 24-hour integrated levels of growth hormone. J. Gerontol. 40 (1985) 2−7.

[18] Frohman, L. A., T. R. Downs, I. J. Clarke et al.: Measurement of growth hormone-releasing hormone and somatostatin in hypothalamic-portal plasma of unanesthetized sheep: spontaneous secretion and response to insulin-induced hypoglycemia. J. Clin. Invest. 86 (1990) 17−24.

[19] Ghigo, E., S. Goffi, E. Arvat at al.: Pyridostigmine partially restores the GH responsiveness to GHRH in normal aging. Acta Endocrinol. 123 (1990) 169−174.

[20] Ghigo, E., S. Goffi, M. Nicolosi et al.: Growth hormone (GH) responsiveness to combined administration of arginine and GH-releasing hormone does not vary with age in man. J. Clin. Endocrinol. Metab. 71 (1990) 1481−1485.

[21] Gil-Ad, I., R. Gurewitz, O. Marcovici et al.: Effect of aging on human plasma growth hormone response to clonidine. Mech. Aging Dev. 27 (1984) 97−100.

[22] Giusti, M., A. Lomeo, G. Marini et al.: Role of aging on growth hormone and prolactin release after growth hormone-releasing hormone and domperidone in man. Horm. Res. 27 (1987) 134−140.

[23] Hartman, M. L., A. C. S. Faria, M. L. Vance et al.: Temporal structure of in vivo growth hormone secretory events in man. Am. J. Physiol. 260(1) (1991) E101−E110.

[24] Hartman, M. L., A. Iranmanesh, M. O. Thorner et al.: Evaluation of pulsatile patterns of growth hormone release in man. AmJHumBiol 5 (1993) 603−614.

[25] Hartman, M. L., J. D. Veldhuis, M. L. Johnson et al.: Augmented growth hormone (GH) secretory burst frequency and amplitude mediate enhanced GH secretion during a two day fast in normal men. J. Clin. Endocrinol. Metabol. 74 (1992) 757–765.

[26] Hendricks, C. M., R. C. Eastman, S. Takeda et al.: Plasma clearance of intravenously administered pituitary human growth hormone: gel filtration studies of heterogeneous components. J. Clin. Endocrinol. Metab. 60 (1985) 864–867.

[27] Hindmarsh, P. C., D. R. Matthews, C. E. Brain: The half-life of exogenous growth hormone after suppression of endogenous growth hormone secretion with somatostatin. Clin. Endocrinol. (Oxf) 30 (1988) 443–450.

[28] Hochberg, Z., P. Hertz, V. Colin et al.: The distal axis of growth hormone in nutritional disorders: GH-binding protein, insulin like growth factor-I (IGF-I) and IGF-I receptors in obesity and anorexia nervosa. Metabolism 41 (1992) 106–112.

[29] Holl, R. W., M. L. Hartman, J. D. Veldhuis et al.: Thirty-second sampling of plasma growth hormone (GH) in man: correlation with sleep stages. J. Clin. Endocrinol. Metab. 72 (1991) 854–861.

[30] Holl, R. W., J. D. Veldhuis, B. Siegler et al.: Half-life of endogenous human growth hormone (GH): diurnal variation and lack of correlation with growth hormone-binding protein (GHBP). Endocrine Society Meeting (1991) (Abstract).

[31] Iovino, M., P. Monteleone, L. Steardo: Repetitive growth hormone-releasing hormone administration restores the attenuated growth hormone (GH) response to GH-releasing hormone testing in normal aging. J. Clin. Endocrinol. Metab. 69 (1989) 910–913.

[32] Iranmanesh, A., G. Lizarralde, M. L. Johnson et al.: Nature of altered growth hormone secretion in hyperthyroidism. J. Clin. Endocrinol. Metab. 72(1) (1991) 108–115.

[33] Iranmanesh, A., G. Lizarralde, J. D. Veldhuis: Age and relative adiposity are specific negative determinants of the frequency and amplitude of GH secretory bursts and the half-life of endogenous GH in healthy men. J. Clin. Endocrinol. Metab. 73 (1991) 1081–1088.

[34] Iranmanesh, A., J. D. Veldhuis: Clinical pathophysiology of the somatotropic (GH) axis in adults. In: J. D. Veldhuis (ed.): Endocrinology and Metabolism Clinics of North America, pp. 783–816. W. B. Saunders, Philadelphia, PA 1993.

[35] Isgaard, J., L. Carlsson, O. G. P. Isaksson et al.: Pulsatile intravenous growth hormone (GH) infusion to hypophysectomized rats increases serum-like growth factor I messenger ribonucleic acid in skeletal tissues more effectively than continuous infusion. Endocrinology 123 (1988) 2605–2610.

[36] Jansson, J. O., K. Albertsson-Wikland, S. Eden et al.: Effect of frequency of growth hormone administration on longitudinal bone growth and body weight in hypophysectomized rats. Acta Physiol. Scand. 114 (1982) 261–265.

[37] Jorgensen, J. O., W. F. Blum, N. Moller et al.: Short-term changes in serum insulin-like growth factors (IGF) and IGF binding protein 3 after different modes of intravenous growth hormone (GH) exposure in GH-deficient patients. J. Clin. Endocrinol. Metab. 72 (1991) 582–587.

[38] Katakami, H., T. R. Downs, L. A. Frohman: Inhibitory effect of hypothalamic medial preoptic area somatostatin on growth hormone-releasing factor in the rat. Endocrinology 123 (1988) 1103–1109.

[39] Kopelman, P. G., K. Noonan: Growth hormone response to low dose intravenous injections of growth hormone releasing factor in obese and normal weight women. Clin. Endocrinology (Oxf) 24 (1986) 157–164.

[40] Kopelman, P. G., K. Noonan, R. Goulton et al.: Impaired growth hormone response to growth hormone releasing factor and insulin-hypoglycemia in obesity. Clin. Endocrinology (Oxf) 23 (1985) 87–94.

[41] Kowarsky, A., R. G. Thompson, C. J. Migeon et al.: Determination of integrated plasma concentration and true secretion rates of human growth hormone. J. Clin. Endocrinol. Metab. **32** (1971) 356−360.

[42] Kraicer, J., M. S. Sheppard, J. Luke et al.: Effect of withdrawal of somatostatin and growth hormone (GH)-releasing factor on GH release **in vitro**. Endocrinology **122** (1988) 1810.

[43] Lang, I., R. Kurz, G. Geyer et al.: The influence of age on human pancreatic growth hormone-releasing hormone stimulated growth hormone secretion. Horm. Metab. Res. **20** (1988) 574−578.

[44] Lumpkin, M. D., S. E. Mulroney, A. Haramati: Inhibition of pulsatile growth hormone (GH) secretion and somatic growth in immature rats with a synthetic GH-releasing factor antagonist. Endocrinology **124** (1989) 1154−1159.

[45] MacGillivray, M. H., L. A. Frohman, J. Doe: Metabolic clearance and production rates of human growth hormone in subjects with normal and abnormal growth. J. Clin. Endocrinol. Metab. **30** (1970) 632−638.

[46] Martha Jr., P. M., K. M. Goorman, R. M. Blizzard et al.: Endogenous growth hormone secretion and clearance rates in normal boys as determined by deconvolution analysis: relationship to age, pubertal status and body mass. J. Clin. Endocrinol. Metab. **74** (1992) 336−344.

[47] Mauras, N., J. D. Veldhuis: Increased hGH production rate after low-dose estrogen therapy in prepubertal girls with Turner's syndrome. Pediatric. Res. **28**(6) (1990) 626−630.

[48] Mode, A., G. Norstedt, B. Simic et al.: Continuous infusion of growth hormone feminizes hepatic steroid metabolism in the rat. Endocrinology **103** (1981) 2103−2108.

[49] Ono, M., N. Miki, H. Demura: Effect of antiserum to rat growth hormone (GH)-releasing factor on physiological GH secretion in the female rat. Endocrinology **129** (1991) 1791−1796.

[50] Owens, D., M. C. Strivastave, C. V. Tompkins et al.: Studies on the metabolic clearance rate, apparent distribution space and plasma half-disappearance time of unlabelled human growth hormone in normal subjects and in patients with liver disease, renal disease, thyroid disease and diabetes mellitus. Eur. J. Clin. Invest. **3** (1973) 284−294.

[51] Parker, M. L., R. D. Vitger, W. H. Daughaday: Studies on human growth hormone. II. The physiological disposition and metabolic fate of human growth hormone in man. J. Clin. Invest. **41** (1962) 262−268.

[52] Pavlou, E. P., S. M. Harman, G. R. Merriam et al.: Responses of growth hormone (GH) and somatomedin-C to GH-releasing hormone in healthy aging men. J. Clin. Endocrinol. Metab. **62** (1986) 595−600.

[53] Pertzelan, A., R. Kerte, B. Bauman et al.: Responsiveness of pituitary GH to GRH 1-44 in juveniles with obesity. Acta Endocrinol. **111** (1986) 151−153.

[54] Prinz, P. N., E. D. Weitzman, G. R. Cunningham et al.: Plasma growth hormone during sleep in young and aged men. J. Gerontol. **38** (1983) 519−524.

[55] Root, A. W., F. A. Oski: Effects of human growth hormone in elderly males. J. Gerontol. **24** (1969) 97−104.

[56] Rosenbaum, M., J. M. Gertner: Metabolic clearance rates of synthetic human growth hormone in children, adult women, and adult men. J. Clin. Endocrinol. Metab. **69** (1989) 821−824.

[57] Rudman, D., M. H. Kutner, M. Rogers et al.: Impaired growth hormone secretion in the adult population: relation to age and adiposity. J. Clin. Invest. **67** (1981) 1361−1369.

[58] Salomon, F., R. C. Cuneo, R. Hesp et al.: The effects of treatment with recombinant human growth hormone on body composition and metabolism in adults with growth hormone deficiency. N. Engl. J. Med. **321** (1989) 1797−1803.

[59] Sato, M., J. Takahara, Y. Fujioka et al.: Physiological role of growth hormone (GH)-releasing factor and somatostatin in the dynamics of GH secretion in adult male rat. Endocrinology **123** (1988) 1928−2933.

[60] Shapiro, B. H., J. N. MacLeod, N. A. Pampori et al.: Signalling elements in the ultradian rhythm of circulating growth hormone regulating expression of sex-dependent forms of hepatic cytochrome P450. Endocrinology **125** (1989) 2935–2944.

[61] Shibasaki, T., K. Shizume, M. Nakahara et al.: Age-related changes in plasma growth hormone response to growth hormone-releasing factor in man. J. Clin. Endocrinol. Metab. **58** (1984) 212–214.

[62] Slowinska-Srzednicka, J., W. Zgliczynski, A. Makowska et al.: An abnormality of the growth hormone/insulin-like growth factor-I axis in women with polycystic ovary syndrome due to coexistent obesity. J. Clin. Endocrinol. Metab. **74** (1992) 1432–1345.

[63] Soya, H., M. Suzuki: Somatostatin rapidly restores rat growth hormone (GH) release response attenuated by prior exposure to human GH-releasing factor **in vitro**. Endocrinoly **122** (1988) 2492–2498.

[64] Sundseth, S. S., J. A. Alberta, D. J. Waxman: Sex-specific, growth hormone-regulated transcription of the cytochrome p450 2C11 and 2C12 genes. J. Biol. Chem. **267**(6) (1992) 3907–3914.

[65] Taylor, A. L., J. L. Finster, D. H. Mintz: Metabolic clearance and production rates of human growth hormone. J. Clin. Invest. **48** (1969) 2349–2358.

[66] Thomas, G. B., J. T. Cummins, H. Francis et al.: Effect of restricted feeding on the relationship between hypophysial portal concentrations of growth hormone (GH)-releasing factor and somatostatin, and jugular concentrations of GH in ovariectomized ewes. Endocrinology **128** (1991) 1151–1158.

[67] Thorner, M. O., M. L. Vance, M. L. Hartman et al.: Physiological role of somatostatin on growth hormone regulation in humans. Metabolism 39 (1990) 40–42.

[68] Ulloa-Aguirre, A., R. M. Blizzard, E. Barcia-Rubi et al.: Testosterone and oxandrolone, a non-aromatizable androgen, specifically amplify the mass and rate of growth hormone (GH) secreted per burst without altering GH secretory burst duration or frequency or the GH half-life. J. Clin. Endocrinol. Metab. **71** (1990) 846–854.

[69] Urban, R. J., W. S. Evans, A. D. Rogol et al.: Contemporary aspects of discrete peak detection algorithms: I. The paradigm of the luteinizing hormone pulse signal in men. Endocr. Rev. **9** (1988) 3–37.

[70] Urban, R. J., J. D. Veldhuis: Hypothalamo-pituitary concomitants of aging. In: J. R. Sowers, J. V. Felicetta (eds.): The Endocrinology of Aging. pp. 41–77. Raven Press, New York 1988.

[71] Veldhuis, J. D.: Dynamics of the hypothalamic pituitary-testicular axis. In: S. S. C. Yen, R. B. Jaffe (eds.): Reproductive Endocrinology. pp. 409–459. W. B. Saunders, Co., Philadelphia, PA 1991.

[72] Veldhuis, J. D., M. L. Carlson, M. L. Johnson: The pituitary gland secretes in bursts: Appraising the nature of glandular secretory impulses by simultaneous multiple-parameter deconvolution of plasma hormone concentrations. Proc. Natl. Acad. Sci. USA **84** (1987) 7686–7690.

[73] Veldhuis, J. D., A. Faria, M. L. Vance et al.: Contemporary tools for the analysis of episodic growth hormone secretion and clearance **in vivo**. Acta Paed. Scand. **347** (1988) 63–82.

[74] Veldhuis, J. D., A. Iranmanesh, K. K. Y. Ho et al.: Dual defects in pulsatile growth hormone secretion and clearance subserve the hyposomatotropism of obesity in man. J. Clin. Endocrinol. Metab. **72** (1991) 51–59.

[75] Veldhuis, J. D., A. Iranmanesh, M. L. Johnson et al.: Twenty-four hour rhythms in plasma concentrations of adenohypophyseal hormones are generated by distinct amplitude and/or frequency modulation of underlying pituitary secretory bursts. J. Clin. Endocrinol. Metab. **71** (1990) 1616–1623.

[76] Veldhuis, J. D., M. L. Johnson: Cluster analysis: A simple, versatile and robust algorithm for endocrine pulse detection. Am. J. Physiol. **250** (1986) E486–E493.

[77] Veldhuis, J. D., M. L. Johnson: Contemporary aspects of deconvolution analysis to appraise **in vivo** neuroendocrine secretory events. In: Frontiers in Neuroendocrinology. pp. 363−383. Raven Press, 1991.

[78] Veldhuis, J. D., M. L. Johnson: Deconvolution analysis of hormone data. Methods in Enzymology **210** (1992) 539−575.

[79] Veldhuis, J. D., M. L. Johnson, L. M. Faunt et al.: Influence of the high-affinity growth hormone (GH)-binding protein on plasma profiles of free and bound GH and on the apparent half-life of GH. J. Clin. Invest. **91** (1993) 629−641.

[80] Veldhuis, J. D., M. L. Johnson, M. J. Wilkowski et al.: Neuroendocrine alterations in the somatotropic axis in chronic renal failure. In: Acta Paed. Scand. pp. 12−22. 1991.

[81] Veldhuis, J. D., G. Lizarralde, A. Iranmanesh: Divergent effects of short-term glucocorticoid excess on the gonadotropic and somatotropic axes in normal men. J. Clin. Endocrinol. Metab. **74** (1992) 96−102.

[82] Veldhuis, J. D., J. F. Sotos, B. M. Sherman et al.: Decreased metabolic clearance of endogenous growth hormone and specific alterations in the pulsatile mode of growth hormone secretion occur in prepubertal girls with Turner's syndrome. J. Clin. Endocrinol. Metab. **73** (1991) 1073−1080.

[83] Vermeulen, A.: Nyctohemeral growth hormone profiles in young and aged men: correlation with somatomedin-C levels. J. Clin. Endocrinol. Metab. **64** (1987) 884−888.

[84] Vizner, B., Z. Reiner, M. Sesko: Effect of L-dopa on growth hormone, glucose, insulin, and cortisol response in obese subjects. Exp. Clin. Endocrinology **81** (1983) 41−48.

[85] Wehrenberg, W. B., A. Baird, S. Y. Ying et al.: The effect of testosterone and estrogen on the pituitary growth hormone response to growth hormone releasing factor. Biol. Reprod. **32** (1985) 369−375.

[86] Weiss, J., M. J. Cronin, M. O. Thorner: Periodic interactions of GH-releasing factor and somatostatin can augment GH release **in vitro**. Am. J. Physiol. **253** (1987) E508−E516.

[87] Weltman, A., J. Y. Weltman, R. Schurrer et al.: Endurance training amplifies the pulsatile release of growth hormone: effects of training intensity. J. Applied Physiology **76**(6) (1992) 2188−2196.

[88] Weltman, J. Y., J. D. Veldhuis, A. Weltman et al.: Reliability of estimates of pulsatile characteristics of luteinizing hormone (LH) and growth hormone (GH) release in women. J. Clin. Endocrinol. Metab. **71** (6) (1990) 1646−1652.

[89] Williams, T., M. Berelowitz, S. N. Joffe: Impaired growth hormone responses to growth hormone-releasing factor in obesity. A pituitary defect reversed with weight reduction. N. Engl. J. Med. **311** (1984) 1403−1407.

[90] Wright, N. M., F. J. Northington, J. D. Miller et al.: Elevated growth hormone secretory rate in premature infants: deconvolution analysis of pulsatile GH secretion in the neonate. Pediatr. Res. **32** (1992) 286−290.

[91] Zadik, Z., S. A. Chalew, R. J. McCarter Jr. et al.: The influence of age on the 24-hour integrated concentration of growth hormone in normal individuals. J. Clin. Endocrinol. Metab. **60** (1985) 513−516.

Growth hormone and aging

Chr. Wüster

1 Introduction

Growth hormone (GH) is secreted in a pulsatile fashion like the gonadotropins or prolactin from the somatotrophic cells of the pituitary gland. It has a strong circadian rhythm, which seems to be regulated by the hypothalamic GH releasing hormone (GHRH) and somatostatin (SRIF). GH stimulates synthesis of the insulin-like growth factor-1 (IGF-1) and some of its binding proteins such as the major IGF-binding-protein-3 (IGFBP-3) in the liver [11]. Serum concentrations of IGF-1 and IGFBP-3 are closely regulated by GH. Their serum concentrations therefore reflect endogenous 24-hour GH-secretion [13]. It is thought that GH also has direct effects on its target organs and thus acts via a dual mechanism [37]: one by direct stimulation on a separate receptor [60] and the other indirect via IGF-1 [93]. Other IGF binding proteins regulate IGF-action like the IGFBP-4 which inhibits the stimulatory effect of IGF-1 on mouse osteoblasts [85]. The GH-receptor belongs to a receptor-superfamily, which includes the prolactin receptor and several cytokine receptors and has a soluble form such as the GH binding protein (GHBP) which might also regulate GH action [16].

2 Effects of GH deficiency (GHD) and GH treatment on different systems

Most of the effects of GH on different systems in adults are known from studies in GHD and from effects seen in patients under treatment with GH. Some effects can also be studied in patients with a pathological increased GH-secretion due to a pituitary tumor: acromegaly or gigantism. Other alternatives are in vitro studies which, however, can never demonstrate the interactions between different systems in vivo, interactions which are particularly multiple in the case of GH-effects.

2.1 Body composition

Body composition is difficult to assess. Many techniques are used, but the different compartments are usually measured only indirectly. Jørgensen et al. [50]

studied 22 GH-deficient adults by means of CT-scanning of the thigh. In the non-GH-treated condition, the distribution of fat and muscle in the thigh was 37% and 63% (as compared with approximately 15% and 85% in healthy subjects). Similarily, Salomon et al. [84] found GH-deficient adults to be over-weight (skinfold thickness) and to have decreased lean body mass (total body potassium method). This was confirmed by our study [99] of adults with GHD due to previous pituitary operations, radiation or tumors. Our results are summarized in Table 1. Other methods used to assess body composition are the

Table 1   Signs and symptoms in 122 patients with growth hormone deficiency due to pituitary tumor, radiation or operation. Adapted from [99] with permission of the author.

Signs and symptoms	Prevalence (in %)
Tiredness, exhaustion and muscle weakness	53
Obesity	40
Hyperlipidemia	77
Hypertriglyceridemia	68
Hypercholesterinemia	68
Hypertension	18
Signs of artherosclerosis (coronary heart disease, stroke)	14
Back pain	36
Decreased spinal bone density (< -1 SD)	57
Decreased radial bone density (< -1 SD)	73
Vertebral fractures	17

bioelectrical impedance (BIA), deuterium oxide dilution (DO) and dual-X-ray-absorptiometry (DXA). The formulas for predicting body composition in normal subjects probably do not apply to GHD adults, as the amount of extra-cellular water in these subjects is smaller than normal and thus leads to an underestimation of lean body mass [58]. Even after correction for these differences, GHD adults had more body fat and less muscle mass compared to age-, sex-, height- and weight-matched controls [10]. BIA and DXA were applied in a subgroup of our patients [104]. The results are shown in Fig. 1. As measured by BIA, GHD patients (males and females) had a significantly ($p < 0.05$) higher percentage of body fat than age- and sex-matched healthy controls. This was confirmed by DXA-measurements in females, but not in males. However when absolute values of body fat (DXA) were related to the individual values of the body mass index (kg/m^2) in males, patients with GHD had higher body fat values compared to healthy controls.

During GH-treatment an average gain in muscle mass of about 3–5 kg and a simultaneous loss of body fat mass of about 2–3 kg can usually be achieved.

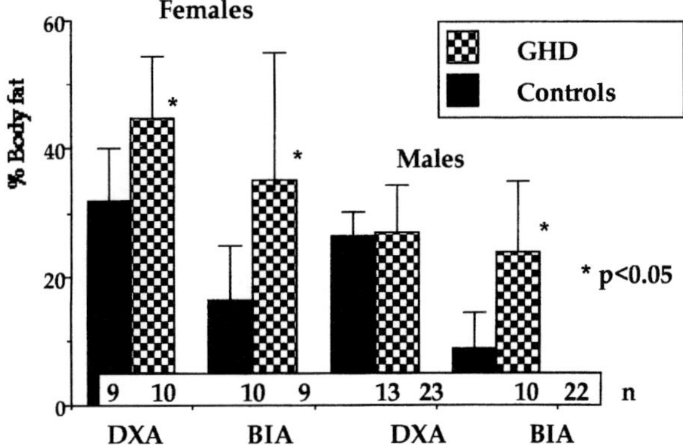

Fig. 1   Percentage of body fat in growth hormone deficient patients (black columns) compared to age- and sex-matched controls (checked columns) measured by bioelectrical impedance (BIA) and dual-X-ray-absorptiometry (DXA). GHD, growth hormone deficiency values are given as means ± SEM. * p < 0.05.

The maximum change in body composition occurs within a few weeks after starting GH treatment. This is possibly due to the sudden decrease in the amount of extra-cellular body water in GHD which affects the formulas used to calculate fat and lean body masses. Using the CT method an 11% increase in lean body mass and a 16% decrease in fat mass was measured [84]. Overall patients gained an average of about 4 kg in body weight after 12–18 months of GH-treatment in this last study.

2.2 Bone metabolism

Effects of GHD on bone metabolism are shown in Table 2. Low bone mass has been measured in children using single-photon-absorptiometry [28, 89]. This method, however, depends on body mass index, which itself is reduced in these children [101]. More recently we have shown low bone mass at the lumbar spine using dual-X-ray-absorptiometry [99]. This was confirmed by Kaufmann et al. showing no difference between isolated and multiple pituitary deficiencies [55]. We furthermore showed an increased prevalence of vertebral fractures indicating osteoporosis in these patients [99]. However Kann et al. have found no difference in the apparent phalangeal ultrasound transmission velocity between GHD and age- and sex-matched controls as a measure of bone elasticity, which is thought to be more related to bone structure than BMD [54]. Possibly a combination of both methods (BMD and elasticity) will give more reliable results. Some of the differences seen between patients with multiple pituitary insufficiencies and isolated GH-deficiency is thought to be due to the additional hormonal replacement therapy. However, no differences between patients receiving L-thyroxine or hydrocortisone and those patients without this substitutional treatment was found in our study [104].

Table 2 Summary of effects of growth hormone deficiency and GH treatment on bone metabolism and bone density. Decr. = decreased, n = normal or no change, incr. = increased, ? = not investigated, iPTH = parathyroid hormone.

	Effects of GH-deficiency	Effects of GH-treatment
Bone formation		
Alkaline phosphatase	decr. − n [72]	n − incr. [72]
Osteocalcin	decr. − n [29, 49, 72]	incr. [10, 49, 63, 64, 72, 86]
Histology	?	incr. [40]
Bone resorption		
Urinary calcium	?	n − incr. [10, 49, 63, 64]
Urinary hydroxyproline	?	incr. [10, 49, 63, 64]
Urinary pyridinolines	n − incr. [86]	n − incr. [86]
Histology	?	incr. [40]
Other markers		
of bone metabolism		
Serum calcium	n	n − incr. [10, 14, 49, 63, 64, 72, 86]
Serum phosphate	n	incr. [10, 14, 49, 63, 64, 72, 86]
Serum iPTH	?	n − incr. [62, 63]
Serum 1,25 vitamin D_3	?	incr. [62]
Bone density	decr. [28, 54, 55, 89, 99]	n [10, 63, 97]
Bone quality	n [54]	?
Vertebral fracture rate	incr. [99]	?

Low serum levels of osteocalcin were measured in GHD patients [29, 72]. However others have shown normal values of osteocalcin [49] and increased urinary pyridinolines as markers of bone resorption in patients with multiple pituitary deficiencies but not with isolated GHD [86].

GH also has effects on mechanical properties and biochemical composition of rat bones [52]. It increased external diameters of long bones whereas the internal diameters were unaffected. In thus improved the mechanical properties of the cortical femur and tibia although bone density, bone collagen content and bone ash weight remained unchanged. These effects might possibly also be explained by the increased weights of the animals [52].

GH undoubtedly stimulates bone turnover [40]. This has been shown by many investigators to be true independent of the state of endogenous GH-secretion: in normal healthy young volunteers [14] and in healthy elderly women [63]. Bone mineral density (BMD) was measured in this last study and showed no change at the spine or femur. These results are consistent with results after short term GH application by the same authors [62]. These effects were reproduced in

GH-deficient adults [10, 49, 72, 86, 97]. An increase in BMD was also not found after GH administration for half a year in GH-deficient adults [97], although numbers of patients and time of treatment periods were insufficient to draw final conclusions with respect to GH-effects on BMD. In elderly men with low IGF-1, a small (1.6%) but significant increase of lumbar BMD without any effects on the hip BMD was measured after 6 months GH-treatment [80]. However this effect on bone mass brains the method of BMD determinations, which has a coefficient of variation of 1−2%. The ineffectiveness of GH in increasing BMD after short GH treatment is possibly due to the simultaneous increase in bone resorption as shown by an increase of urinary pyridinolines [86]. GH also has stimulatory effects on bone resorption as shown more recently in osteoclasts cultures in vitro [66], however it is not known whether this is a direct effect or is mediated by a "coupling factor" like IL-6 [90]. Possibly GH is only able to reconstitute bone mass lost in GH-deficiency by increasing a hypothetical skeletal set point of BMD without having any further BMD-increasing effects beyond this point.

2.3 Energy, carbohydrate, lipid and protein metabolism

GH treatment increased the basal metabolic rate by 16% [84]. Fasting plasma glucose, insulin, C-peptide and the ratio of insulin: C-peptide increased with active treatment [84]. There was no change in HbA_1 [84]. In GHD adults, GH treatment prevents the development of hypoglycemia during starving. It has been reported that GHD patients have a prevalence of hyperlipidemia (Table 1). The lipolytic effect of GH is well documented [36]. GH has been shown to promote a redistribution of adipose tissue from an abdominal to a more peripheral (from android to gynoid) distribution [104] and to decrease lipogenesis [75]. Plasma total cholesterol decreased on GH-treatment, while triglycerides remained unchanged. There was a rise in plasma free fatty acids and glycerol in the GH-treated group [84]. Furthermore GH has been shown to play an important role in the regulation of hepatic LDL receptors and thus might be necessary for the control of plasma LDL levels [6, 77]. These authors showed that the estrogen-induced increase of the hepatic LDL receptor number in hypophysectomized rats was strongly exaggerated by addition of GH. This LDL-receptor stimulation was also shown in liver specimens of gall-stone patients pre-treated with GH before operation. This was accompanied by a 25% decrease in serum cholesterol. The effects of GH on the LDL-receptor were of the same magnitude as a 3 week treatment with hypolipidemic drugs such as pravastatin or simvastatin [6].

2.4 Muscle strength and exercise capacity

Cuneo et al. have shown reduced muscle strength using a dynamometer [23−25]. This was already suggested by Ranke in an early note [73]. We confirmed these complaints of increased lethargy and muscle fatigue in a larger group of patients [99]. GH-treatment improves muscle functions leading to a better exercise capacity as evaluated by a standard ergometer [50]. During the exercise tests, maximum oxygen uptake increased by 24% between zero and 6 months and this was associated with a 20% increase in power output (149W to 177W) [24]. Studies with 15N-glycine showed an increase in exercise capacity and muscle strength, and an increased rate of protein synthesis during long-term GH supplementation of GHD adults [10].

2.5 Cardiovascular effects

GH-treatment seems to improve cardiac function in healthy and GHD subjects [50, 94]. However GHD patients do not show any pathological values in echocardiography. After GH-treatment no changes in left ventricular wall thickness were seen, but in increased left ventricular end-diastolic volume by 2% and stroke volume by 6.1%. No effect on blood pressure was recorded apart from one patient in the English study who became hypertensive, which normalized after dose reduction [84].

2.6 Renal effects and effects on the renin-aldosterone system

GH is known to increase the glomerular filtration rate and renal plasma flow in healthy subjects [19]. In GHD both parameters were found to be reduced [32, 50]. GH-treatment normalized renal function. In patients with intact adrenal function, plasma renin activity increased during GH-treatment while aldosterone levels remained unchanged [92]. Serum concentrations of the atrial natriuretic peptide decreased [68]. Another marked GH-effect is seen on sodium retention leading to fluid retention up to frank edema in patients under high dose of GH [92]. In young healthy adults without GHD, administration of GH resulted in a reduction of urinary sodium excretion and urine volume, but not osmolality. Plasma renin activity increased, as did serum aldosterone. Plasma osmolality and arginine vasopressin levels did not change [44].

2.7 Psychological and social aspects

Adults with GHD who were treated with GH during childhood have shown a low percentage of marriage and a high risk of unemployment [27, 48]. McGauley conducted a study comparing the psychological well-being of adults with GHD to age- and sex-matched normals [64]. GHD patients perceived themselves as being more labile, more socially isolated and less energetic than did the controls. They furthermore regarded themselves as having a poorer level of general health, less self-control and less vitality and they experienced more anxiety. A significant improvement in the self-assessed quality of life was found after GH supplementation. These results were confirmed by Degerblad et al. [28]. Longer and larger studies using GH supplementation in GHD will have to be conducted in order to show its effects on the rate of unemployment, which might not be due GHD itself, but rather to the fact that these are patients with chronic illness.

2.8 Mortality

In a retrospective analysis of 333 patients with hypopituitarism diagnosed over a period of 30 years, Rosen et al. suggested a shortened life-span, especially due to deaths form cardiovascular diseases [74]. On the other hand, these patients seem to suffer and die from cancer to a lesser degree than expected. The mortality risk was increased irrespective of whether hypopituitarism was due to pituitary adenoma or secondary to other causes.

2.9 Effects on the immune system

GH leads indirectly to harm the immune system via a reduced activity of natural killer cells [56]. GH effects on the immune system will indirectly influence bone metabolism by a variety of cytokines such as TNFα and a number of interleukins. A possible direct or indirect action (i.e. via immune cells) of GH on osteoclasts should be considered and is being investigated.

2.10 Effects on the reproductive system

Endogenous GH regulates the intraovarian IGF-1 system [2]. IGF-1 is produced by the ovaries themselves after stimulation with GH. Ovaries show the third highest level of IGF-1 gene expression in the rat [2]. In humans the granulosa cells however seem to be a site of IGF-2 rather then IGF-1 gene expression. IGF-1 can increase the differentiated phenotypic expression of the developing granulosa cell [1]. Furthermore, IGF-1 is capable of augmenting FSH-supported progesterone and estrogen biosynthesis as well as the FSH-mediated acquisition of LH receptors. Like in bone, the IGF-1 system in the granulosa cell is regulated by IGF-binding proteins locally. Furthermore, it has been suggested that IGF-1 is important for the selection of the dominant follicle, assuming timely and selective activation of the IGF-1 system in "chosen" follicles [2]. An autocrine/paracrine IGF-1 system seems to be an important component of the estrogen-induced uterine proliferative response [70]. This of course may represent one of a number of autocrine/paracrine growth factor systems operative in the uterus.

IGF-1 and GH play an important role in the development of Sertoli cells and Leydig cells [82]. Reduced semen quality has been reported in men with isolated GH-deficiency. However, GH-treatment in males does not seem to improve this defect [82, 87]. Schreiner et al. have furthermore presented that there was no change in the size of the prostate or any effect on prostate fluid after GH-treatment. However, it is necessary to investigate the potential effects of improving the sexual life of patients with GHD as it seems to be an important part of one's quality of life and little is known in this field.

3 GH and nutrition

Patients with obesity show an attenuated GH response to most stimuli of GH-secretion [57, 98]. However serum IGF-1 levels are higher in obese patients than in patients with normal weight. It is thought that low GH secretion in obesity is due to increased IGF-1. Short term GH administration was effective in decreasing the loss of lean body mass in patients on diets, but fat loss was not accelerated [21].

Fasting results in an increase of GH pulse frequency, amplitude, and interpulse GH levels and a decline of IGF-1 after 5 days [43]. Patients with anorexia nervosa show similar results [18]. Patients with kwashiokor or marasmus have high levels of GH in the presence of low insulin, albumin and amino acid levels [7]. They returned to normal after refeeding.

In critically ill patients with sepsis, the basal secretory rates of GH were higher, but had similar pulse frequencies [76]. Post-operatively IGF-1 levels decrease as they do in other catabolic states. The paradox of high GH and low IGF-1 suggests that these patients have "GH resistance". GH treatment of patients with catabolic states have already shown good evidence that nitrogen balance can be improved. Furthermore, GH treatment improved the efficacy of parenteral nutrition in a double-blind placebo controlled study [106]. However, high concentrations of GH have been required in some studies in order to demonstrate an anabolic effect. These doses can lead to significant insulin resistance and in some cases to overt hyperglycemia. In other studies it was shown that catabolic normal volunteers become refractory to the anabolic effects of GH after periods of 4−5 weeks of treatment. Furthermore the degree of anabolic response seems to be a limitation of the use of GH in catabolic states as it depends on the degree of catabolism. The anabolic response of GH in severely catabolic patients is attenuated. Therefore IGF-1 has been used instead to overcome this problem and first success has been achieved [21]. However, in order to get a substantial suppression of protein breakdown a substantial increase of IGF-1 is needed. The danger of hypoglycemia is therefore necessary and high infusion rates of glucose are needed. Further studies are needed to solve the many open questions in this field.

4 GH and aging

4.1 Physiological changes

GH-secretion declines with age [65, 78], a phenomenon called "somatopause". The characteristics of this age-dependent change are shown in Table 3. This

Table 3   Characteristics of "somatopause".

Decreased central cholinergic tonus →↑ somatostatin
Decreased hypothalamic GHRH mRNA expression
Decreased expression of pituitary GHRH receptors
Decreased GH response after GHRH
Decreased IGF-1 response after GH- or GHRH
Decreased number of GH pulses
Decreased GH- and GHBP serum concentrations
Decreased GH half-life time
Decreased IGF-1- and IGFBP-3 concentrations
Decreased GH secretion after sports activity

decline in endogenous GH-secretion has been attributed to the inhibitory action of increased secretions of somatostatin [96], as also shown in aging rats [17]. This might be due to the general decrease of the cholinergic nerves with aging, as hypothalamic GHRH-mRNA expression decreases with age, as do the expression of pituitary GHRH receptors. The stimulated GH response to any stimulatory agent decreases with age [15, 35, 53, 59, 69, 88]. The same applies to the integrated 24-hour GH values [3, 45, 34, 105] and to IGF-1 concentrations in serum [9, 22, 41, 81]. Serum IGFBP-3 levels have been shown to be closely related to 24-hour GH secretion in children [12]. However we were unable to demonstrate an age-related decline in serum IGFBP-3 levels in healthy females (Fig. 2, lower panel) [100, 102]. These determinations were based on subjects up to the age of 65, thus it is possible that the age-related decline was missed.

Reduced physical activity has been suggested as being responsible for the low GH values in the elderly. However it was recently shown in the findings of Pyka et al. [83] that elderly people are not able to increase their endogenous GH secretion by exercise as younger people are. Furthermore, this group treated elderly women with a vigorous exercise program for one year and did not find an increase of IGF-1 serum levels compared to a non-exercising age- and sex-matched group [62]. Thus reduced exercise levels in the elderly do not explain the effects seen with "somatopause".

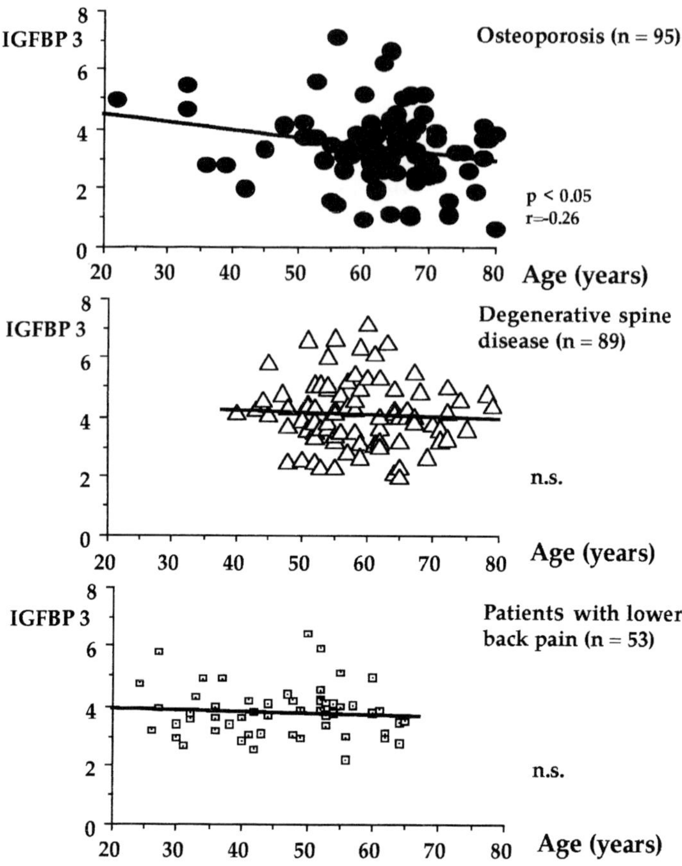

Fig. 2   Serum concentrations of IGFBP-3 [13] in females with primary postmenopausal osteoporosis (top), with degenerative spine disease (middle) and in controls (bottom) in relation to age. A significant age-related decline of serum IGFBP-3 was seen only in patients with established osteoporosis as shown by the presence of vertebral fractures, but not in patients with osteoarthritis or patients with back pain but without spinal radiological changes.

Menopause itself has also been suggested to cause changes seen during "somatopause", as estrogen has a strong effect on GH secretion. Serum 24-hour GH levels as well as serum IGF-1 decreases after menopause [26, 45, 95]. Oral estrogen replacement inhibits hepatic IGF-1 synthesis and re-increases GH secretion through reduced feedback inhibition. However, reduced GH secretion in menopause is not explained by estrogen deficiency alone, since GH secretion is not restored by the attainment of physiological E_2 levels using the transdermal route. As some signs of "somatopause" are also seen in aging men without any relation to their testosterone levels, it is questionable whether sex steroid deficiency alone explains the age-related decrease in GH secretion. Possibly a similar relationship between sex steroids and GH as that seen in puberty is taking place in "somatopause". In puberty estrogens have an additive effect to GH on bone growth, whereas testosterone seems to have a potentiating effect [47]. Whether the reverse is true in age-related changes has yet to be investigated.

4.2 Effects of GH-treatment in healthy subjects and in old age

GH has been given to young males [14] and to healthy elderly people [63, 64] for short periods. The effects were similar to those seen in GHD and described above. Rudman et al. [80] treated elderly men with low IGF-1 levels with GH for one year. They also reported on the known effects of GH on muscle and fat mass. Furthermore, they showed a significant increase in lumbar bone mineral density which was not seen at any other sites (hip and radius) and might be due to a statistical problem, as no multivariance analysis was shown in their report. It is doubtful whether this effect can be reproduced and whether it would last for a longer period. Recently Marcus et al. reported a study of GH treatment in healthy postmenopausal elderly women. They did not see any significant effect on BMD after one year of treatment [63]. Thus it seems that GH has its greatest potential in patients with GHD or low IGF-1. The possibility that it could restore all deficiencies seen with age and act as a fountain of youth seems to be unrealistic.

5 GH-secretion and effects of GH-treatment in osteoporosis

GH-secretion in patients with osteoporosis was found to be reduced after stimulation with L-arginine in comparison to patients with osteoarthrosis [30]. We showed low serum IGF-1, IGF-2 and IGFBP-3 as measured by radioimmunoassays [13] in 98 females with postmenopausal osteoporosis compared to 59 normal subjects and 91 patients with degenerative bone disease [102]. Results are shown in Fig. 2 for IGFBP-3. Similar results were measured in males with osteoporosis, and serum IGF-1 and IGFBP-3 concentrations were positively correlated with lumbar BMD in osteoporotic patients. Comparable results have been found by others for IGF-1 [61, 71]. Patients with osteoarthrosis seemed to have higher values [102]. This is consistent with results from studies on IGF-2 concentrations in bones from patients with osteoarthrosis [67]. Treatment of osteoporotic patients with GH has not been successful in the past although an increase of serum and histology markers of bone turnover has been achieved [3−5]. The studies, however, contained few patients, and again treatment periods were too short to study vertebral fracture rates, the gold standard in the determination of efficacy of an antiosteoporotic drug. New studies combine PTH- and GH-treatment in males with osteoporosis [39].

6 Risks and side effects of GH treatment

Side effects of GH substitution in GHD and of GH treatment in elderly men with low IGF-1 were very rare [84]. Initially arthralgias can be observed, which is resolved by lowering the dose. The same applies to edema and muscle pain occasionally seen. Hypertension and hyperglycemia can be a problem, although hypertension is resolved by dose reduction. Blood glucose only increased when looking at the mean of the whole group and was not accompanied by a significant increase in glycosylated hemoglobin. Only when using high doses, as needed in catabolism, can overt hyperglycemia be a problem. The question of cancer induction is open. As can be seen from epidemiological studies, there is a decreased probability of cancer death in GHD patients. Thus it is expected that this decreased cancer prevalence will be "normalized". Whether cancer will increase probably depends on the dose of GH used and the levels of IGF-1 achieved.

7 Summary and conclusions

GH is a potent anabolic hormone for almost all systems including bone and calcium metabolism. Patients with GHD have signs and symptoms summarized in Table 1. It has been suggested that this is a new syndrome by Sönksen et al. [92]. Most of the deficiencies can be restored by substitution of GH. However the results of ongoing larger and longer studies have to be seen in order to draw final conclusions on the effects of GH on the risk for arteriosclerosis and subsequent mortality due to cardiovascular diseases. Furthermore, the results of these studies will show the effects on bone mineral density and fracture rates due to osteoporosis fractures. Some patients with established osteoporosis and vertebral fractures seem to suffer from GHD. A combination of the effects of menopause and "somatopause" as a reason for osteoporosis has been hypothesized and is schematized in Figure 3. Treatment of osteoporosis with GH alone

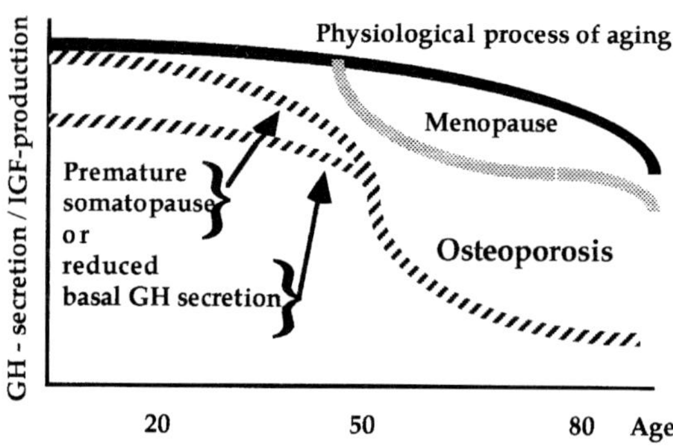

Fig. 3   Hypothetical model of the involvement of "somatopause" in the pathogenesis of osteoporosis.

or in combination with calcitonin has not been successful in the past. Studies with more patients over several years to investigate effects of GH treatment on the vertebral fracture rate are missing. As GH seems to reverse some signs of old age such as muscle weakness and reduced exercise capacity, one might speculate the GH could prevent the occurrence of hip fractures in elderly people. This however has to be discussed looking at the ethical and financial aspects of GH-treatment in the elderly.

Acknowledgements

I wish to thank Ulrike Rehn, Ulrike Härle, Sylke Schlemilch and Ellen Slenczka for their active work during their theses, Johannes Erdmann and Sigrid Butz for their clinical work with the GHD patients, Marina Götz for determinations of bone density, Werner Blum, University Childrens' Hospital Tübingen for the opportunity to use his radioimmunoassays, Reinhard Ziegler for his critical advice and helpful support and Andreas Attanasio (Eli Lilly, Bad Homburg) and Heinz Steinkamp (Pharmacia, Erlangen) for their financial and intellectual support.

References

[1] Adashi, E. Y., C. E. Resnick, A. J. Dércole et al.: Insulin-like growth factors as intraovarian regulators of granulosa cell growth and function. Endocr. rev. 6 (1985) 400−420.

[2] Adashi, E. Y., C. E. Resnick, E. R. Hernandez et al.: The Intraovarian IGF-1 system. In: E. M. Spencer (ed.): Modern concepts of insulin-like growth factors, 267−274. Elsevier Science Publishing New York−Amsterdam−London−Tokyo 1991.

[3] Aloia, J. F., I. Zanzi, K. Ellis et al.: Effects of growth hormone in osteoporosis. J. Clin. Endocr. Metab. 43 (1976) 922−999.

[4] Aloia, J. F., A. Vaswani, A. Kapoor et al.: Treatment of osteoporosis with calcitonin with and without growth hormone. Metabolism 34 (1985) 124−131.

[5] Aloia, J. E., A. Vaswani, P. J. Meunier et al.: Coherence treatment of postmenopausal osteoporosis with growth hormone and calcitonin. Calcif. Tissue Int. 40 (1987) 253−259.

[6] Angelin, B., M. Rudling, H. Olivecrona et al.: Effects of growth hormone on low-density lipoprotein metabolism. Acta Pædiatr. Suppl. 383 (1992) 67−68.

[7] Becker, D. J.: The endocrine responses to protein calorie malnutrition. Ann. Rev. Nutr. 3 (1983) 187−212.

[8] Bengtsson, B. Å., R. J. M. Brummer, S. Edén et al.: Effects of growth hormone on fat mass and fat distribution. Acta Pådiatr. Suppl. 383 (1992) 62−65.

[9] Bennett, A. E., H. W. Wahner, B. L. Riggs et al.: Insulin-like growth factors I and II: aging and bone density in women. J. Clin. Endocrin. Metabol. 59 (1984) 701−704.

[10] Binnerts, A., G. R. Swart, J. H. P. Wilson et al.: The effect of growth hormone administration in growth hormone deficient adults on bone, protein, carbohydrate and lipid homeostasis, as well as on body composition. Clin. Endocrinology 37 (1992) 79−87.

[11] Blum, W. F., M. B. Ranke, K. Kietzmann et al.: A specific radioimmunoassay for the growth hormone (GH)-dependent somatomedin-binding protein: its use for diagnosis of GH deficiency. J. Clin. Endocrinol. Metab. 70 (1990 a) 1292−1298.

[12] Blum, W. F., M. B. Ranke: Use of insulin-like growth factor-binding protein 3 for the evaluation of growth disorders. Horm. Res. 33 (Suppl. 4) (1990 b) 31−37.

[13] Blum, W. F., K. Albertsson-Wikland, S. Rosberg et al.: Insulin-like growth factor binding protein 3 (IGFBP-3) reflects spontaneous growth hormone (GH) secretion. Horm. Res. 33 (Suppl. 3) (1990 c) 3−9.

[14] Brixen, K., H. K. Nielsen, L. Mosekilde et al.: A short course of recombinant human growth hormone treatment stimulates osteoblasts and activates bone remodeling in normal human volunteers. J. Bone Miner Res. 5 (1990) 609−618.

[15] Carlson, H. E., J. C. Gilin, P. Gorden et al.: Absence of sleep-related growth hormone peaks in aged normal subjects and in acromegaly. J. Clin. Endocrinol. Metab. 34 (1972) 1102−1105.

[16] Carlsson, B., S. Eden, A. Nilsson et al.: Expression and physiological significance of growth hormone receptors and growth hormone binding protein in rat and man. Acta Pediatr. Scand. (Suppl.) 379 (1991) 70−76.

[17] Casad, R. C., R. C. Adelman: Aging enhances inhibitory action of somatostatin in rat pancreas. Endocrinology 130 (1992) 2420−2421.

[18] Casanuev, A. F. F., L. Villnueva, L. A. Cabranes et al.: Cholinergic mediation of growth hormone secretion elicited by arginine, clonidine, and physical activity in man. J. Clin. Endocrinol. Metabol. 59 (1987) 526−530.

[19] Christiansen, J. S., J. Gammelgaard, H. Ørskov et al.: Kidney function and size in normal subjects before and during growth hormone treatment for one week. Eur. J. Clin. Invest. 11 (1981) 487−490.

[20] Clemmons, D. R., D. K. Snyder, R. Williams et al.: Growth hormone administration conserves lean body mass during dietary restriction in obese subjects. J. Clin. Endocrinol. Metab. 64 (1987) 878−883.

[21] Clemmons, D. R.: Editorial: Role of insulin-like growth factor-1 in reversing catabolism. J. Clin. Endocrinol. Metabol. 75 (1992) 1183−1185.

[22] Copeland, K. C., R. B. Colletti, J. T. Devlin et al.: The relationship between insulin-like growth factor-I, adiposity and aging. Metabolism 39 (1990) 584−587.

[23] Cuneo, R. C., F. Salomon, C. M. Wiles et al.: Skeletal muscle performance in adults with growth hormone deficiency. Horm. Res. 33 (Suppl. 4) (1990) 55−60.

[24] Cuneo, R. C., F. Salomon, C. M. Wiles et al.: Growth hormone treatment in growth hormone deficient adults. I. Effects on muscle mass and strength. J. Appl. Physiol. 70 (1991) 688−694.

[25] Cuneo, R. C., F. Salomon, C. M. Wiles et al.: Growth hormone treatment in growth hormone deficient adults. II. Effects on exercise performance. J. Appl. Physiol. 70 (1991) 695−700.

[26] Dawson-Hughes, B., D. Stern, J. Goldman et al.: Regulation of growth hormone and somatomedin-C secretion in postmenopausal women: effect of physiological estrogen replacement. J. Clin. Endocrinol. Metab. 63 (1986) 424−432.

[27] Dean, J. H., T. L. McTaggert, D. G. Fish et al.: The education, vocational and maritial status of growth hormone-deficient adults treated with growth hormone during childhood. Am. J. Dis. Child. 39 (1985) 1105−1110.

[28] Degerblad, M., O. Almkvist, R. Grunditz et al.: Physical and psychological capabilities during substitution therapy with recombinant growth hormone in adults with growth hormone deficiency. Acta Endocrinol. (Copenh.) 123 (1990) 185−193.

[29] Delmas, P. D., P. Chatelain, L. Malaval et al.: Serum bone Gla-protein in growth hormone deficient children. J. Bone Mineral. Res. 1 (1986) 333−338.

[30] Dequeker, J., A. Burssens, R. Bouillon: Dynamics of growth hormone secretion in patients with osteoporosis and in patients with osteoarthrosis. Hormone Res. **16** (1982) 353−356.

[31] Ernst, M., E. R. Froesch: Growth hormone dependent stimulation of osteoblast-like cells in serum free cultures via local synthesis of insulin-like growth factor I. Biochem. Biophys. Res. Commun. **151** (1988) 142−147.

[32] Falkheden, T.: Renal function following hypophysectomy in man. Acta Endocrinol. (Copenh.) **42** (1963) 571−578.

[33] Finkelstein, J. W., H. P. Rolfwarg, R. M. Boyar et al.: Age-related changes in the twenty-four hour spontaneous secretion of growth hormone. J. Clin. Endocrinol. Metabol. **35** (1972) 665−670.

[34] Florini, J. R., P. N. Prinz, M. V. Vittelo: Somatomedin C levels in healthy young and old men: relationship tp peak and 24 hour integrated levels of growth hormone. J. gerontol. **40** (1985) 2−10.

[35] Franchimont, P.: Effects of repetitive administration of growth hormone-releasing hormone on growth hormone secretion, insulin-like growth factor I and bone metabolism in postmenopausal women. Acta Endocrinol. **120** (1989) 121−128.

[36] Goodman, H. M., J. Schwartz: Growth hormone and lipid metabolism. In: E. Knobil, W. H. Sayer (eds.): Handbook of physiology. Vol. 4, part 2. Washington DC: Am. Physiol. Soc., pp. 211−232, 1974.

[37] Green, H., M. Morikawa, T. Nixon: A dual effector theory of growth hormone action. Differentiation **29** (1985) 195−198.

[38] Häger, A.: Should adults with growth hormone deficiency be maintained on growth hormone substitution therapy? Acta Pædiatr. Scand. Suppl. **362** (1989) 72-75.

[39] Harms, H. M., S. König, P. R. Wüstermann et al.: Knochenstoffwechselparameter bei Patienten mit Osteoporose unter Therapie mit humanem Parathormon-(1-38)(hPTH1-38) und rekombinantem Wachstumshormon (rhGH). In: C. Wüster, R. Raue, R. Ziegler (Hrsg.): Osteologie '92, S. 29. Merges, Heidelberg 1992.

[40] Harris, E. H., R. P. Heaney, J. Jowsey et al.: Growth hormone: the effect of skeletal renewal in the adult dog. I. morphometric studies. Calcif. Tissue Res. **10** (1972) 1−13.

[41] Hattori, N., H. Kurahachi, K. Ikekubo et al.: Effects of sex and age on serum GH binding protein levels in normal adults. Clin. Endocrinol. **35** (1991) 295−297.

[42] Ho, K. Y., W. S. Evans, R. M. Blizzard et al.: Effects of sex and age on the 24-hour profile of growth hormone secretion in man: importance of endogenous estradiol concentrations. J. Clin. Endocrinol. Metabol. **64** (1987) 51−58.

[43] Ho, K. Y., J. D. Veldhuis, M. L. Johnson et al.: Fasting enhances growth hormone secretion and amplifies the complex rhythm of growth hormone secretion in man. J. Clin. Invest. **81** (1988) 968−975.

[44] Ho, K. Y., A. J. Weissberger: The antinatriuretic action of biosynthetic human growth hormone in man involves activation of the renin-angotensin system. Metabolism **39** (1990a) 133−137.

[45] Ho, K. Y., A. J. Weissberger: Secretory patterns of growth hormone according to sex and age. Horm. Res. **33** (Suppl. 4) (1990b) 7−11.

[46] Isaksson, D. G. P., A. Lindahl, A. Nilsson et al.: Mechanism of the stimulatory effect of growth hormone on longitudinal bone growth. Endocr. Rev. **8** (1987) 426−438.

[47] Jansson, J. O., S. Edén, O. Isaksson: Sexual dimorphism in the control of growth hormone secretion. Endocrine reviews **6** (1985) 128−150.

[48] Job, J. C., J. Chicaud, J. E. Toublanc: Le devenir long terme des nains hypophysaires traités par l'hormone de croissance. Arch. Fr. Pediatr. **45** (1988) 169−173.

[49] Johansen, J. S., S. A. Pedersen, J. O. L. Jørgensen et al.: Effects of growth hormone (GH) on plasma Bone Gla protein in GH-deficient adults. J. Clin. Endocrinol. Metab. 70 (1990) 916–919.

[50] Jørgensen, J. O. L., S. A. Pederson, L. Thuesen et al.: Benefitial effects of growth hormone treatment in GH-deficient adults. Lancet i (1989) 1221–1225.

[51] Jørgensen, J. O. L., W. F. Blum, N. Moller et al.: Circadian patterns of serum insulin-like growth factor (IGF) I and IGF binding protein 3 in growth hormone deficient patients and age- and sex-matched normal subjects. Acta Endocrinol. (Copenh.) 123 (1990) 257–262.

[52] Jørgensen, P. H., B. Bak, T. T. Andreassen: Mechanical properties and biochemical composition of rat cortical femur and tibia after long-term treatment with biosynthetic human growth hormone. Bone 12 (1991) 353–359.

[53] Kalk, W. J.: Growth hormone response to insulin hypoglycemia in the elderly. J. Gerontol. 28 (1973) 431–433.

[54] Kann, P., B. Piepkorn, A. Pfützner et al.: Bone quality in growth hormone deficient adults. Presentation at the International meeting on growth hormone deficiency in adults, Stockholm, November 20–21, 1992.

[55] Kaufman, J. M., P. Taelman, A. Vermeulen et al.: Bone mineral status in growth hormone-deficient males with isolated and multiple pituitary deficiencies of childhood onset. J. Clin. Endocrinol. Metab. 74 (1992) 118–123.

[56] Kiees, W., H. Doerr, E. Eisl et al.: Lymphocyte subsets and natural killer activity in growth hormone deficiency. N. Engl. J. Med. 314 (1986) 321 (letter).

[57] Kopelman, P. G., K. Noonan, R. Goulton et al.: Impaired growth hormone response to growth hormone releasing hormone release from rat pituitary in vitro. Clin. Endocrinology 23 (1985) 87–94.

[58] Lamberts, S. W. J., N. K. Valk, A. Binnerts: The use of growth hormone in adults: a changing scene. Clin. Endocrinol. 37 (1992) 111–115.

[59] Lang, I., G. Schernthaner, P. Pietschmann et al.: Effects of sex and age on growth hormone response to growth hormone-releasing hormone in healthy individuals. J. Clin. Endocrinol. Metab. 65 (1987) 535–540.

[60] Leung, D. W., S. A. Spencer, G. Cachines et al.: Growth hormone receptor and serum binding protein: purification, cloning and expression. Nature 330 (1987) 537–543.

[61] Ljunghall, S., F. A. Karlsson, O. Kämpe et al.: Is circulating IGF-1 a determinant for male osteoporosis? J. Bone Min. Res. 6 (Suppl. 1) (1991) 223.

[62] Marcus, R., G. Butterfield, L. Holloway et al.: Effects of short term administration of recombinant human growth hormone to elderly people. J. Clin. Endocrinol. Metab. 70 (1990) 519–527.

[63] Marcus, R.: Growth hormone – a fountain of youth? Presentation at the German investigator meeting of the Kabi GH study. Benzheim/Auerbach 28. 9. 1992.

[64] McGauley, G. A., R. C. Cuneo, F. Salomon et al.: Psychological well-being before and after growth hormone treatment in adults with growth hormone deficiency. Horm. Res. 33 (Suppl. 4) (1990) 52–54.

[65] Meites, J.: Neuroendocrine biomarkers of aging in the rat. Exp. Gerontol. 23 (1988) 349–358.

[66] Mochizuki, H., Y. Hakeda, N. Wakatsuki et al.: Insulin-like growth factor-I supports formation and activation of osteoclasts. Endocrinology 131 (1992) 1075–1080.

[67] Mohan, S., J. Dequeker, R. Van Den Eyned et al.: Increased IGF-I and IGF-II in bone from patients with osteoarthritis. J. Bone Min. Res. 6 (Suppl. 1) (1991) 131.

[68] Møller, J., J. O. L. Jørgensen, N. Møller et al.: Expansion of extracellular volume and suppression of atrial natriuretic peptide after growth hormone administration in normal man. J. Clin. Endocrinol. Metabol. 72 (1991) 768–772.

[69] Muggeo, M., D. Fedele, A. Tiengo et al.: Human growth hormone and cortisol responses to insulin stimulation in aging. J. Gerontol. 30 (1975) 546−551.

[70] Murphy, L. J.: The uterine insulin-like growth factor system. In: E. M. Spencer (ed.): Modern concepts of insulin-like growth factors, 275−284. Elsevier Science Publishing New York−Amsterdam−London−Tokyo 1991.

[71] Nakamura, T., T. Hosoi, Y. Mizuno et al.: Clinical significance of serum levels of insulin like growth factors as bone metabolic markers in postmenopausal women. Bone Mineral. 17 (Suppl. 1) (1992) 170.

[72] Nielsen, H. K., J. O. L. Jørgensen, K. Brixen et al.: Serum osteocalcin and bone isoenzyme alkaline phosphatase in growth-hormone-deficient patients: dose-response studies with biosynthetic human GH. Calcif. Tiss. Intern. 46 (1991) 82−87.

[73] Ranke, M. B.: A note on adults with growth hormone deficiency. Acta Pædiatr. Scand. (Suppl.) 331 (1987) 80−82.

[74] Rosen, T., B. A. Bengtsson: Premature mortality due to cardiovascular disease in hypopituitarism. Lancet 336 (1990) 285−288.

[75] Rosenbaum, M., J. M. Gertner, R. Leibel: Effects of systemic growth hormone (GH) administration on regional adipose tissue distribution and metabolism in GH-deficient children. J. Clin. Endocr. Metab. 69 (1989) 1274−1281.

[76] Ross, R. J. M., C. R. Buchanan: Growth hormone secretion: its regulation and the influence of nutrional factors. Nutrion research Reviews 3 (1990) 143−162.

[77] Rudling, M., G. Norstedt, H. Olivecrona et al.: Importance of growth hormone for the induction of hepatic low density lipoprotein receptors. Proc. Natl. Acad. Sci. 89 (1992) 6983−6987.

[78] Rudman, D., M. H. Kutner, C. M. Rogers et al.: Impaired growth hormone secretion in the adult population: relation to age and adiposity. J. Clin. Invest. 67 (1981) 1361−1369.

[79] Rudman, D.: Growth hormone, body composition, and aging. J. Am. Geriatr. Soc. 33 (1985) 800−807.

[80] Rudman, D., A. G. Feller, H. S. Nagraj et al.: Effects of growth hormone in men over 60 years old. N. Engl. J. Med. 323 (1990) 1−6.

[81] Pavlov, E. P., S. M. Harman, G. R. Merriam et al.: Response of growth hormone (GH) and somatomedin-C to GH-releasing hormone in healthy aging men. J. Clin. Endocrinol. Metabol. 62 (1986) 595−600.

[82] Pedersen, S. A., J. O. Jørgensen, J. S. Christiansen et al.: Growth hormone and reproduction: Reduced semen quality in men previously treated for growth hormone deficiency. In: H. Frisch, M. O. Thorner (eds.): Hormonal regulation of growth Serono Symposia Publications 58, 1989, 273−282. Raven Press New York.

[83] Pyka, G., R. A. Wiswell, R. Marcus: Age-dependent effect of resistance exercise on growth hormone secretion in people. J. Clin. Endocrinol. Metab. 75 (1992) 404−407.

[84] Salomon, F., R. C. Cuneo, R. Hesp et al.: The effects of treatment with recombinant human growth hormone on body composition and metabolism in adults with growth hormone deficiency. N. Engl. J. Med. 321 (1989) 1797−1803.

[85] Scharla, S. H., D. D. Strong, S. Mohan et al.: 1,25-dihydroxyvitamin D_3 differentially regulates the production of insulin-like growth factor I (IGF-I) and IgF-binding protein-4 in mouse osteoblasts. Endocrinology 129 (1991) 3139−3146.

[86] Schlemmer, A., J. S. Johansen, S. A. Pedersen et al.: The effect of growth hormone (GH) therapy on urinary pyridinoline cross-links in GH-deficient adults. Clin. Endocrinology 35 (1991) 471−476.

[87] Schreiner, T., Effects of GH replacement therapy on genito-urinary systems. Presentation at the Third International Meeting on Clinical research on growth hormone deficiency in adults. Stockholm November 20−21, 1992.

[88] Shibaski, T., K. Shizume, M. Nakhara et al.: Age-related changes in plasma growth hormone response to growth hormone-releasing hormone in man. J. Clin. Endocrinol. Metabol. **58** (1984) 212–214.

[89] Shore, R. M., R. W. Chesney, R. B. Mazess et al.: Bone mineral status in growth hormone deficiency. J. Pediatrics **96** (1980) 393–396.

[90] Slootweg, M. C., W. W. Most, E. Van Beek et al.: Osteoclast formation together with interleukin-6 production in mouse long bones in increased by insulin-like growth factor-I. J. Endocrinology **132** (1992) 433–438.

[91] Slootweg, M.: Growth hormone and bone. Hormone Res **25** (1993) 335–43.

[92] Sönksen, P. H., R. C. Cuneo, F. Salomon et al.: Growth hormone therapy in adults with growth hormone deficiency. Acta Pædiatr. Scand. [Suppl.] **379** (1991) 139–146.

[93] Stracke, H., A. Schulz, R. Rossol et al.: Effect of growth hormone on osteoblasts and demonstration of somatomedin C/IGF I in bone organ culture. Acta Endocrinol. (Copenh.) **107** (1984) 16–24.

[94] Thuesen, I., J. S. Christiansen, K. E. Sørensen et al.: Increased myocardial contractility following growth hormone administration in normal man. An echocardiographic study. Dan. Med. Bull. **35** (1988) 193–196.

[95] Weissberger, A. J., K. K. Y. Ho, L. Lazarius: Constrating effects of oral and transdermal routed of estrogen replacement therapy on 24-hour growth hormone (GH) secretion, insulin-like growth factor I, and GH-binding protein in postmenopausal women. J. Clin. Endocrinol. Metab. **72** (1991) 374–381.

[96] Wehrenberg, W. B.: Physiological role of somatocrinin and somatostatin in the regulation of growth hormone secretion. Biochem. Biophys. Res. Comm. **109** (1975) 562–567.

[97] Whitehead, H. M., C. Boreham, E. M. Mcilrath et al.: Growth hormone treatment of adults with growth hormone deficiency: results of a 13-month placebo controlled cross-over study. Clin. Endocrinology **36** (1992) 45–52.

[98] Williams, T., M. Berelowitz, S. N. Joffe et al.: Impaired growth hormone responses to growth hormone releasing hormone factor in obesity: a pituitary defect reversed with weight reduction. N. Engl. J. Med. **311** (1984) 1403–1407.

[99] Wüster, Chr., E. Slenczka, R. Ziegler: Erhöhte Prävalenz von Osteoporose und Arteriosklerose bei konventionell substituierter Hypophysenvorderlappeninsuffizienz: Bedarf einer zusätzlichen Wachstumshormonsubstitution? Klin. Wochenschr. **69** (1991) 769–773.

[100] Wüster, Chr., W. Blum, S. Schlemilch et al.: Decreased serum levels of IGF-binding protein (IGFBP-3) in osteoporosis. J. Bone Min. Res. **6** (Suppl. 1) (1991) 107.

[101] Wüster, Chr., G. Duckeck, A. Ugurel et al.: Bone Mineral Content of Spine and Forearm in Osteoporosis and in German Normals: Influences Of Sex, Age and Anthropometric Parameters. Eur. J. Clin. Invest. **22** (1992) 366–370.

[102] Wüster, Chr., W. F. Blum, S. Schlemilch et al.: Decreased serum levels of insulin like growth factors 1 and 2 and IGF binding protein-3 in patients with osteoporosis. J. Intern. Med. **234** (1993) 249–255.

[103] Wüster, Chr.: Growth hormone and bone. Acta Endocrinologica **128** (Suppl. 2) (1993) 14–18.

[104] Zachmann, F. F., D. Tassinari, R. Thakker et al.: Anthropometric measurements in patients with growth hormone deficiency before treatment with human growth hormone. Eur. J. Pediatr. **133** (1980) 227–282.

[105] Zadik, Z., S. A. Chalew, Z. Gilula et al.: Reproducibility of growth hormone testing procedures: a comparison between 24-hour integrated concentration and pharmacological stimulation. J. Clin. Endocrinol. Metab. **71** (1990) 1127–1130.

[106] Ziegler, T. R., J. L. Rombeau, L. S. Young et al.: Recombinant human growth hormone enhances the metabolic efficacy of parenteral nutrition: a double-blind, randomized controlled study. J. Clin. Endocrinol. Metab. **74** (1992) 865–873.

Diagnosis and treatment of thyroid diseases in the aging

W. A. Scherbaum, G. H. Scholz

1 Introduction

1.1 Pathological anatomy of the aging thyroid

The thyroid decreases in weight and becomes fibrotic with age. The follicular size and the colloid content decrease and there is atrophy of glandular epithelium. The histology of the senile thyroid is characterized by an increase of interfollicular connective tissue with the formation of large fibrous areas surrounding scattered glandular islands (for review see: Felicetta [23]).

The human thyroid becomes more nodular with age: ninety percent of women above the age of seventy and sixty percent of men above eighty have thyroid nodules. This prevalence of multinodular goiter seems to be independent of iodine supplementation. In one large postmortem study, solid nodules were detected in more than 80% of females and more than 50% of males over age 70 and in virtually all individuals over age 90 [54].

Many elderly individuals have an enlarged thyroid gland. An ultrasound study of 569 subjects above the age of 60 from the general population in an iodine-deficient area in Germany showed a goiter prevalence of 54.2% in females and 22.5% in males [39]. About 18% of the individuals had one or more thyroid nodules.

It is debatable whether the thyroid volume increases with age [34], or whether an involution of the gland occurs.

2 Changes in biochemical parameters

2.1 Iodine metabolism

There is no doubt that iodine metabolism is altered during aging. The 24-hour radioactive iodine uptake progressively decreases in subjects from 50 to 90 years of age [27]. In people over age 80, the absolute iodine uptake was reported to be only 60% of the uptake measured in subjects below 40 years of age. The iodine uptake for females was about 75% of that for males [32]. There is also an age-dependent decrease in thyroid iodine clearance, a decrease in thyroid hormone synthesis, and a decrease in thyroid hormone metabolism.

2.2 Thyroxine (T4)

In spite of profound changes in thyroxine metabolism in old age, serum T4 levels were reported to be unaltered in the normal aged [71, 87, 33, 42], but seem to decrease progressively with age in other studies [38, 1]. There is an age-related decrease in both thyroid hormone synthesis and peripheral thyroid hormone metabolism. The half life of circulating thyroxine increases from 7 days in younger people to 9 days in individuals above the age of eighty. Turnover kinetics have shown the daily production of thyroxine to decrease by 20 µg in old age [36]. T4 output from the thyroid gland and T4 distribution space, as well as its metabolic clearance rate, also substantially decrease with age [31]. The level of thyroxine-binding globulin was reported to be uneffected by advancing age [52, 33].

2.3 Triiodothyronine (T3)

T3 levels and free T3 indices are slightly decreased in healthy elderly individuals. This applies to men above age 60 and women above age 80 [87, 71, 33, 85, 67]. Above the age of 100 years (centenarians), free T3 is significantly lower than in younger age groups [50]. It seems that males have significantly lower T3 values than females [86]. The lower T3 in the elderly may be due to a decrease in the T3 production rate [32] with an unchanged or even increased metabolic clearance of T3. Reverse T3 was reported to be higher in the elderly [86] and in the centenarians [50]. In contrast to other investigators, Kabadi and Rosman [42] did not find any significant alterations in T3 resin uptake, serum T3 and rT3 when carefully selected euthyroid healthy untreated adults of different age groups were compared. A recent study of a large group of middle-aged and younger adults supported this result. There was no significant difference between these age groups for T3 and estimated free T3 [37].

2.4 Thyrotropin (TSH) secretion

TSH secretion is probably decreased in the elderly [85, 50]. The normal diurnal variation of TSH levels, with a nocturnal acrophase and an afternoon nadir, as well as the pulsatile nature of TSH release, are preserved in elderly men and women [85, 67], (Fig. 1), and the thyroid retains its capacity to respond to acute increases in TSH concentrations [85].

During repeated TRH stimulation, the TSH response fatigues earlier in elderly subjects [84]. In one well-designed study, the overall 24-hour TSH secretion in older men was approximately 50% lower than in young men, and the pituitary was found to be less responsive to TRH in the elderly. However, the chronobiological modulation was preserved and the TRH-induced serum T3 and T4 levels

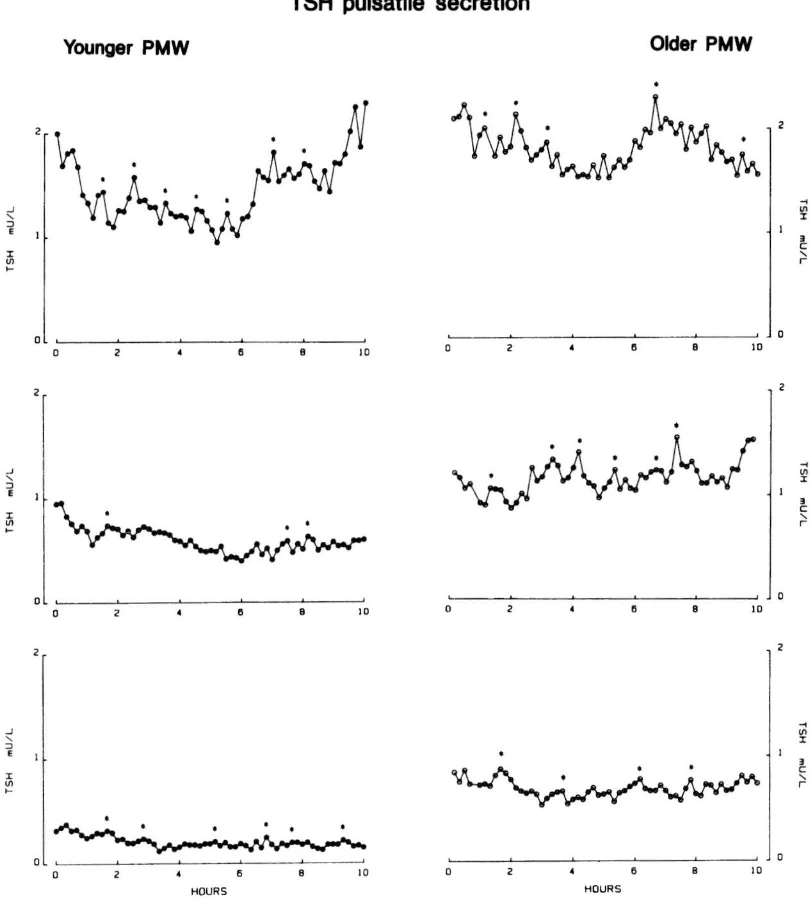

Fig. 1   TSH secretory profiles of younger (closed symbols) and three older (open symbols) post-menopausal women (PMW). Asterisks denote significant TSH pulses, as determined by Cluster analysis.

were of similar magnitude in both groups [85]. These alterations were attributed to an adaptation to the reduced need for thyroid hormones in old age.

However, the results of the measurement of TSH levels in healthy older people are controversial. In a large group of elderly patients, the basal TSH level did not differ significantly from their middle aged offspring. The mean TSH in elderly women was slightly but significantly lower than that in middle-aged women. However, when euthyroid women with positive antithyroid antibodies were excluded, the difference was not significant. There was no difference in mean TSH between younger and older men [37]. In a study of 93 individuals aged 60 to 104 years without clinical evidence of thyroid dysfunction, significantly higher TSH levels were found in comparison to middle-aged normal adults [86]. The same observation was made in another study where younger and older individuals were compared for basal TSH [33]. Elevated TSH in the presence of normal peripheral thyroid hormone levels may reflect a true increase in the prevalence of subclinical hypothyroidism with aging. A decreased TSH level or a blunted TSH response to thyrotropin-releasing hormone may be due to subclinical hyperthyroidism.

2.5 Prevalence and significance of abnormally low or high thyrotropin (TSH) concentrations in the elderly

A decreased TSH level and a suppressed TRH test can be observed in some normal elderly individuals so that these criteria alone are not always useful in establishing thyrotoxicosis in old age [78, 57]. In 55 virtually euthyroid hospitalized patients, abnormalities were found only in patients over 75 years with a less marked and frequently delayed increase of TSH, with a maintained T3 response 120 min after TRH and a normal basal TSH level [16]. In the Whickham survey where 2779 people were studied, TSH levels did not vary with age in males, but increased markedly in females after the age of 45 years. This rise was virtually abolished when individuals with thyroid antibodies were excluded [83].

In an unselected population of individuals above the age of 60 years, the overall prevalence of thyroid deficiency, as demonstrated by a clearly elevated serum TSH level, was 4.4%. In women, hypothyroidism (5.9%) was more frequent than in men (2.3%). Only 40% of those with clearly elevated TSH levels had low T4 levels and the remainder had serum T4 levels in the lower half of the normal range [70].

In a survey of 1210 individuals over 60 years of age in the general population in the U. K., elevated TSH levels were found in 11.6% of females and 2.9% of males. TSH levels were below normal in 6.3% of females and 5.5% of males. At initial testing, 18 individuals were hypothyroid and one was hyperthyroid. Of the 73 individuals with elevated TSH but normal free T4 who were followed up for 12 months, 13 developed hypothyroidism with low free T4 levels, TSH returned to normal in 4 and serum TSH continued to be high in 56. Of the 50 subjects with low but detectable TSH, 38 returned to normal, whereas of those with undetectable TSH 14 remained low at a follow up of 12 months [57].

Thus we can conclude from these studies:
(1) thyroid dysfunction is common in old age
(2) thyroid dysfunction is more frequent in women than in men
(3) the rate of progression to hypothyroidism is very slow
(4) TSH alone does not always reflect the actual thyroid state in the elderly but seems to be a helpful indicator together with the peripheral hormones.

3 Thyroid autoimmunity in the elderly

3.1 Chronic lymphocytic thyroiditis (autoimmune thyroiditis) in the elderly

Autoimmune thyroiditis is one of the most frequent autoimmune diseases in humans. It is characterized by a chronic lymphocytic infiltration in the thyroid and a high concentration of antimicrosomal (equivalent to anti-thyroperoxidase, TPO) and antithyroglobulin antibodies in the blood. It may lead to a clinically relevant atrophy of the gland [20].

The prevalence of circulating antithyroid antibodies constantly increases up to the age of 80 years and then seems to decline in the very old [51]. In a recent study of 342 elderly subjects with a mean age of 80, Roti [68] found a prevalence of thyroid microsomal antibodies (anti-TPO) of 2.3% in men and 10.2% in women. Regarding positive antimicrosomal and antithyroglobulin antibodies, the highest prevalence of anti-TPO was found in patients aged 10 to 19 years in a Japanese population [1] with a progressive reduction in older groups, suggesting that at least in Japan an association of anti-TPO with Hashimoto's thyroiditis is less prevalent in aged patients. These results are difficult to interpret, especially in elderly patients, because the levels of antibodies to TPO do not directly correlate with thyroid function. In spite of clearly demonstrable thyroid failure with elevated serum TSH, antimicrosomal antibodies were not found in 33% of the patients over age 60. Of those with positive antimicrosomal antibodies, 60% did not have thyroid failure [69]. High antimicrosomal antibody titres in combination with an elevated TSH seem to have value for prediction of future hypothyroidism [73].

In one study, eight of twenty-six elderly individuals with TSH levels above 4 mU/ml developed hypothyroidism over a period of four years. All patients with initial TSH levels above 20 mU/ml and 80% of subjects with thyroid microsomal antibody titres above 1 : 1600 developed hypothyroidism over a four year period [76]. However, the prevalence of positive antithyroid antibody levels is highly variable between populations [63].

Histological studies at autopsy revealed lymphocytic infiltrates in the thyroids of elderly individuals. Focal lymphocytic thyroiditis was observed in 20% of the glands [17]. In a large collection of 1826 representative thyroid sections of Japanese subjects, there was a significantly higher overall prevalence of lymphocytic infiltration in females (22.2%) than in males (13.9%), but in the females the prevalence rates reached a maximum during the fourth decade (23.2%) and did not further increase with age. In the parallel investigation of thyroid sections of 810 British subjects, the prevalence was 42.5% in females and 19.4% in males. The prevalence of thyroiditis in females increased from the sixth decade onwards, reaching 50% in those aged over 70 years [56]. In another histopathological autopsy study, focal lymphocytic infiltration was found in 17.2% of thyroid glands of 169 individuals ranging from 63 to 97 years of age, without clear relationship between the prevalence of focal lymphocytic infiltration and age [45].

3.2 Graves' disease

Graves' disease is characterized by hyperthyroidism in the presence of antibodies stimulating the TSH-receptor. In aged patients Graves' disease seems to be less severe because the responsiveness of the thyrocyte to abnormal stimulation may be reduced [1].

One of the problems strongly related to Graves' disease is endocrine ophthalmopathy. In a survey of 101 consecutive patients with this disease, a highly significant relationship was found between age and ophthalmopathy index, indicating the severity of ophthalmopathy. The female to male ratio of Graves' endocrinopathy is about 4 to 1, but males with Graves' thyrotoxicosis above the age of 60 are at an increased risk of developing severe eye disease [58].

3.3 Effects of iodine supplementation on thyroid function and morphology in the elderly

Studying autopsy protocols of the years 1949/50 and 1978/79, Gerber [28] found that in 1949/1950 the thyroids of younger adults were significantly lighter than those of older subjects, probably as a result of the goiter prophylaxis with iodized salt, introduced in 1923 in Switzerland. In 1978/79 the thyroids were only half the weight of those in the years 1949/1950 and goiter prevalence had decreased to the same degree.

This positive result is accompanied by the problem that iodine supplementation has different effects on young and older patients with thyroid disorders. In a recent survey the prevalence of toxic goiter and Graves' disease was studied in two countries with high (Iceland) and low average iodine intake (Denmark). In Denmark, patients above 50 years of age had no endemic goiter but a higher prevalence of multinodular toxic goiter and single toxic adenoma. In Iceland, the prevalence of Graves' disease was significantly higher than in Denmark, particularly in the younger age group [47].

4 Nonthyroidal illness and malnutrition

Severe nonthyroidal illness such as infection, renal disease, heart failure, malignancy, trauma, burns, major surgery and trauma, as well as malnutrition, alter biochemical parameters of thyroid function [4, 29].

Nonthyroidal illness leads to a decrease in serum T3 and an increase of reverse T3 (rT3); depending on the severity of the disease, serum T4 may also fall. In a study of 190 hospitalized patients age 60 and older, Simons [74] found abnormalities of thyroid function tests in 73%. The severity of illness was a stronger predictor of the T3 level than was age. Mortality is inversely correlated with serum T4 levels [76]. In severe non-thyroidal illness, serum TSH may also be lowered and the TSH response to TRH blunted. Therefore, a normal TSH level or a normal TSH response to TRH rules out the diagnosis of hyperthyroidism, but does not completely exclude the existence of primary hypothyroidism.

Malnutrition in elderly individuals is probably more frequent than expected. Starvation changes T3-production and may lead to a 50%−60% decrease of serum T3 [13]. In a recent study, the relationship between nutrient intake and thyroid hormone status in free-living elderly individuals was analyzed. The free T3 level was lower in the subjects with poor health status, whereas high rT3 levels were associated with low energy intake [29].

5 Multinodular goiter and thyroid cancer in old age

As indicated above, the human thyroid becomes more nodular with age, even in areas with sufficient iodine supply. Attempts to suppress the growth or to reduce the size of euthyroid multinodular goiters in old age by T4 replacement therapy may result in iatrogenic hyperthyroidism since functionally autonomous areas are often present in such goiters. Only careful ultrasound assessment and follow-up monitoring may reveal the appearance of a new nodule which requires further investigation, for example by fine needle aspiration biopsy. The presence of tumor-associated symptoms such as hoarseness or dysphagia are usually signs of progressive and invasive thyroid malignancies. An expanding neck mass visibly grown within a few weeks to a few months, with or without enlarged cervical lymph nodes, may indicate anaplastic thyroid carcinoma or lymphoma of the thyroid. The frequencies of both tumors increase with age.

In patients over age 80, up to half of the thyroid carcinomas are anaplastic, whereas differentiated thyroid carcinomas prevail in young age groups [12, 3, 43]. In spite of a lower frequency of differentiated carcinomas in the elderly, the prognosis of these carcinomas is often poor, with a 10 year survival rate of only about 60% compared with 96% in young patients after total thyroidectomy followed by radioiodine ablation [61]. This might be explained by an increasing probability of DNA aneuploidy with increasing age [41, 40].

Thyroid lymphoma, although a rare disease, is most commonly seen in elderly women and often associated with Hashimoto's thyroiditis, which may be considered as a predisposing condition [35]. In 245 patients, mostly elderly women, with lymphoproliferative disorders involving the thyroid gland, the lymphoma was nearly always associated with an underlying lymphocytic thyroiditis [12]. The lymphoma, which is often derived from B-cells, can be treated by chemotherapy and/or by total gross resection of the thyroid and radiation therapy, when it is restricted to the gland [8, 75].

In general, two types of changes were described in Calcitonin producing cells (C-cells) during aging. One may represent an involutional process and the second is a hyperplastic (micronodular) lesion, which appears to increase with age. Often an infiltration by lymphocytes is encountered [5]. C-cell carcinoma or medullary thyroid carcinoma is mainly diagnosed at a younger age. The hereditary form is diagnosed at young age, whereas nonhereditary forms increase in number with age. About 80% of the hereditary tumors were found in the age group below 20 years, whereas only 4% were diagnosed above the age of 60 [60]. One of the negative prognostic parameters is old age at onset of C-cell carcinoma [62].

6 Hypothyroidism in the elderly

The prevalence of hypothyroidism increases with age and approaches five per cent in some studies [63]. An autoimmune cause accounts for approximately 90% of hypothyroidism in adults, in Japan mostly due to Hashimoto's thyroiditis [2]. Some of the initially euthyroid patients progress to hypothyroidism with time, so that the prevalence of hypothyroidism is higher in elderly patients.

The clinical features of hypothyroidism are similar in old age and in the young, but the signs and symptoms of hypothyroidism such as dry skin, cold intolerance, heart failure, mental failure, paraesthesia, anemia and others are frequently mistakenly attributed to the aging process. Misdiagnosis is especially frequent in elderly individuals without an apparent goiter [86] and may lead to considerable delay in adequate treatment (Fig. 2). The risk of developing hypothyroidism increases with age and is especially high in patients who were previously treated with thyroid surgery or radioiodine or with antithyroid drugs.

Thyroxine replacement therapy should be initiated carefully in old age, especially when there is associated ischaemic heart disease. The initial recommended dose is 25 μg per day with an increase of 25 μg per day at 4- to 6-week intervals with ECG monitoring. There is considerable variability in the individual

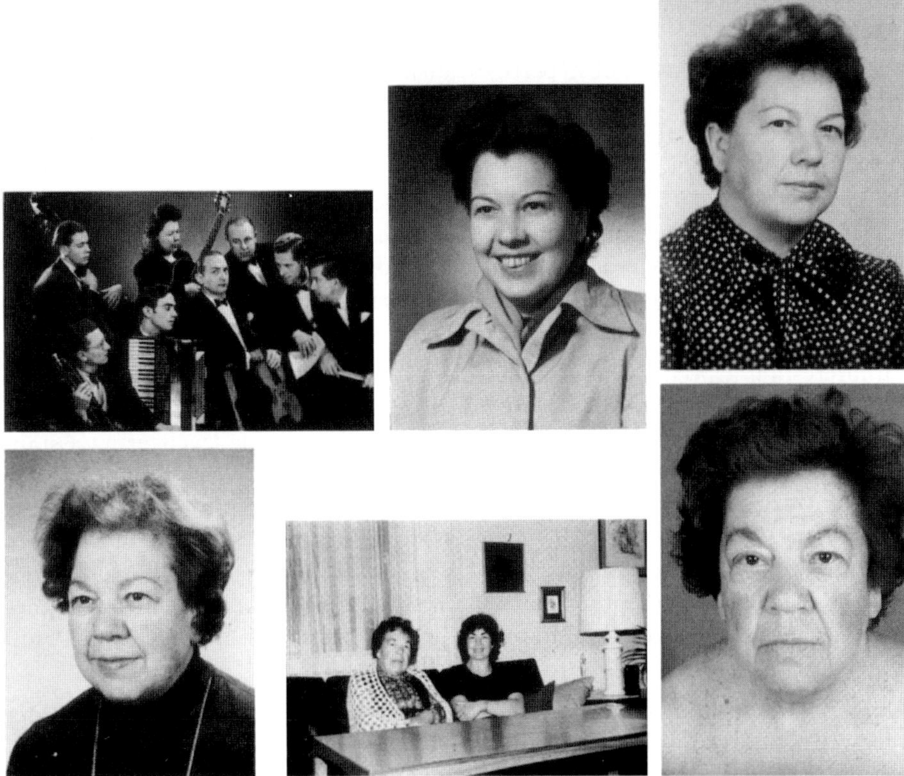

Fig. 2   65 year-old female with severe primary myxoedema. The slow development of hypothyroidism in autoimmune thyroiditis is shown here over a period of 32 years. In 1953 she was an active member of a music band (upper left). The patient presented with full-blown myxoedema and undetectable serum T4 levels in 1985 (lower right).

requirement of T4 to keep basal serum TSH levels in the normal range. The appropriate dose should be titrated out on the basis of normalized TSH levels and the clinical situation of the patient [79]. In case of ischaemic heart disease the T4 replacement should not lead to or aggravate cardiac complications.

7 Hyperthyroidism in the elderly

The prevalence of hyperthyroidism is markedly increased in individuals over the age of 60 [64, 14]. In elderly patients, the most common cause of hyperthyroidism is toxic multinodular goiter (68%) followed by solitary thyroid nodules (16%) and Graves' disease (16%) [7].

The signs and symptoms of hyperthyroidism may be obscured in the elderly. A great portion of patients have oligo- or monosymptomatic hyperthyroidism which may be misdiagnosed without the aid of thyroid hormone and thyrotropin determinations. Cardiovascular disorders are often the first and sometimes the only symptom [7]. Over age 75, the average number of symptoms is 2 and in some cases hyperthyroidism can be present without any specific clinical symptoms [82]. Even thyrotoxic crisis can be overlooked if "nonspecific" symptoms such as headache, cachexia and psychosis are dominant. Adequate management can completely resolve the problem, even in patients over 70 [72].

An interesting aspect of the age-dependence of clinical symptoms was recently evaluated [81]. An attempt was made to relate clinical expression of Graves' disease and Plummer's disease to age and thyroid hormone levels using a standardized clinical score and multiple regression analyses. It was found that patients with Graves' disease tend to have more signs and symptoms than patients with Plummers' disease. After controlling for diagnosis and FT4 index there was no age dependence of the clinical score. The commonly accepted age-dependence of clinical symptoms is thought to be due to the well known higher prevalence of Graves' disease among younger age groups in contrast to Plummer's disease [81].

A comparison of signs and symptoms of hyperthyroidism in younger and older age groups is given in Fig. 3.

It is apparent that sympathetic signs are blunted whereas cardiac symptoms prevail in old age. Muscle weakness as well as psychiatric symptoms are often present in thyrotoxicosis in the elderly.

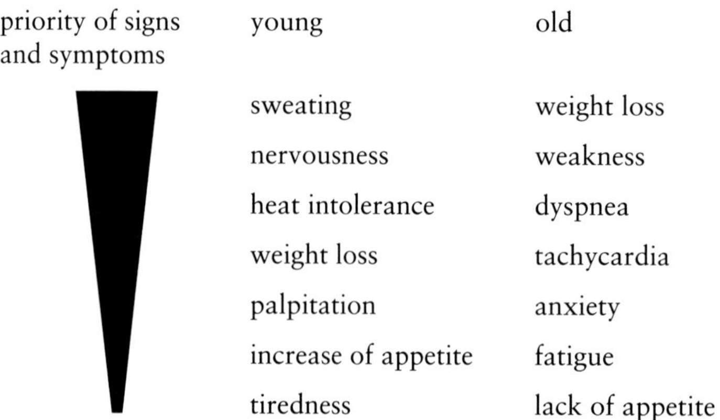

Fig. 3   Clinical signs of hyperthyroidism in young and elderly individuals.

8 Thyroid hormones and the heart

The heart is very sensitive to thyroid hormones. Even small changes in thyroid hormone concentration may influence its metabolism and performance [6, 19, 49]. Palpitations, anginal symptoms, atrial arrhythmias, limitations in exercise tolerance, congestive heart failure and even a tendency to thrombotic events are reported to occur as a result of hyperthyroidism, especially in elderly patients [22, 11, 10, 15, 53].

Successful treatment may reverse most of the symptoms [77, 46] and can also restore exercise tolerance [49]. The older heart, which often has a reduced coronary reserve with a relatively lower oxygen supply, has only a limited capacity to adapt to the local and systemic changes in metabolism and hemodynamics induced by thyroid hormone excess. Early diagnosis of thyroid disease and prompt treatment with antithyroid medication, as well as supportive therapy with nonselective β-blockers such as propranolol, are the main tools in managing cardiac complications.

9 Thyroid hormones and bone metabolism

An appropriate concentration of circulating thyroid hormones is necessary to prevent bone loss. Recent studies have suggested that patients receiving thyroxine may be at increased risk of bone loss [59]. This problem deserves special attention because of the above-mentioned increase in the prevalence of hypothyroidism, as well as hyperthyroidism due to thyrotoxic goiters especially in elderly women.

In a short-term study of 17 postmenopausal women with subclinical hypothyroidism, randomly assigned to thyroxine treatment or no treatment, the bone mineral density of the wrist and the lumbar spine was measured before and after about 14 months of treatment. No change in bone density was found [66]. In a study of 78 postmenopausal women who had been treated with thyroxine for primary hypothyroidism for a minimum of 5 years, a small decrease in forearm bone mineral density was found in the TSH suppressed patients, but the difference from the control group was not statistically significant [30].

Another study compared the bone mineral density of premenopausal and postmenopausal women after long term thyroxine treatment or hyperthyroidism in remission. A significant negative correlation between the cumulative dose of L-T4 and bone mineral density was found only in the postmenopausal women with substantial bone loss in the areas consisting predominantly of trabecular bone, for example the lumbar spine and Ward's triangle [9].

The situation is slightly different in females after total thyroidectomy for thyroid carcinoma. To suppress TSH secretion, higher thyroxine doses are required. Under these conditions, biochemical parameters such as alkaline phosphatase and osteocalcin, as well as urinary excretion of hydroxyproline, are significantly elevated, suggesting high bone turnover [44]. Such suppressive therapy can be associated with substantial bone loss in the lumbar spine, femoral neck and trochanter [44] or in the midshaft radius and the proximal scanning site of the distal forearm, as well as in the calcaneus, of postmenopausal but not premenopausal women [48]. In the latter study, there was no change in the bone mineral density of the lumbar spine, in accordance with other well controlled studies of bone mineral density in trabecular bone in comparable groups of patients [26, 80, 21, 24].

Endogenous subclinical or clinical hyperthyroidism is known to cause significant changes in specific parameters of bone metabolism [55]. In a cross sectional study, premenopausal and postmenopausal women with non-toxic nodular goiter, subclinical hyperthyroidism and toxic solitary autonomous thyroid nodule, were evaluated for changes in bone mineral density in lumbar spine, femoral neck and midshaft of the radius [25]. Lumbar spine density was decreased only in the toxic nodular goiter group, and this decrease was more marked in the postmenopausal women. The bone mineral density at the femoral neck and midshaft radius was slightly, but significantly, decreased only in the postmenopausal women, whereas in both groups, among women with a toxic solitary nodule the midshaft radius was also severely effected. According to these results, cortical bone seems to be a preferential site of action of excess thyroid hormone.

Thyroid hormone induced changes in bone mineral density seem to be reversible. In 15 premenopausal and postmenopausal women with active Graves' thyrotoxicosis, biochemical parameters of bone turnover and bone mineral density in the lumbar spine and femoral neck and trochanter were measured before and after 12 months of antithyroid therapy. There was no significant change in femoral neck and femoral trochanter, but a significant increase in bone mineral density of the lumbar spine. The severity of thyrotoxicosis was independently associated with the percentage increment in lumbar spine bone mineral density after therapy [18].

Summarizing these results, the risk of postmenopausal women developing osteoporosis following substitutive thyroxin therapy is low, compared with the advantage of a normal endocrine status. TSH-suppressive thyroxine therapy after total thyroidectomy because of thyroid carcinoma might have some negative effects on bone, but seems to affect only postmenopausal women with additional risk factors for osteoporosis.

There is no doubt that thyrotoxicosis has detrimental effects on bone metabolism, but successful treatment may even reverse bone loss.

10 Concluding remarks

Thyroid structure and function change with age. The thyroid gland becomes more nodular and iodine uptake, thyroid hormone synthesis and metabolism are decreased in the elderly. In spite of these changes, serum T4 levels are usually not altered. Serum T3 is sometimes decreased, especially in men above 60 and women above 80 years. A decreased basal TSH level and a slightly reduced TSH response to TRH can be observed, but the pulsatile nature of the TSH release and the chronobiological modulation is preserved with a nocturnal acrophase and an afternoon nadir.

Thyroid dysfunction is common in old age and is more frequent in women than in men, but the progression is slow. Thyroid autoimmunity is common in the elderly. An increased prevalence of anti-TPO antibodies and a high prevalence of focal lymphocytic infiltration is found in older individuals but there is no clear relationship between these histopathological findings and age. Hashimoto's thyroiditis is the main cause of hypothyroidism in the elderly. In the elderly hypothyroidism presents with the same clinical signs and symptoms as in the young, but it is often misdiagnosed because the clinical features are ascribed to the aging process. Graves' disease is rather less frequent in the elderly and then causes less severe hyperthyroidism. The most common cause of hyperthyroidism in the elderly is toxic multinodular goiter especially in areas of iodine deficiency. In spite of the markedly increased prevalence of this important disorder, it may be overlooked. The clinical symptomatology is frequently reduced to one or two "nonspecific" symptoms which can mislead the clinician. In clinically unclear situations, the determination of basal TSH and the free T4 values are reliable diagnostic parameters.

In the interpretation of test results, nonthyroidal illness and medical treatment have to be considered as potential modulators of thyroid function, thyroid hormone binding and metabolism.

Thyroid cancer, especially anaplastic thyroid carcinomas, prevail in elderly patients. It is crucial to distinguish this from lymphoma, which is most commonly seen in elderly women with underlying autoimmune thyroiditis.

Hypo- and hyperthyroidism, whether caused by a disease or by medication, have a more marked influence on the heart and bones in the elderly. The clinical importance of thyroid dysfunction in the elderly population should stimulate each clinician to draw attention to early diagnosis and treatment.

References

[1] Aizawa, T., M. Ishihara, K. Hashizume et al.: Age-related changes of thyroid function and immunologic abnormalities in patients with hyperthyroidism due to Graves' disease. J. Am. Geriatr. Soc. 37 (1989) 944−948.

[2] Amino, N.: Autoimmunity and hypothyroidism. Bailliere's Clin. Endocrinol. Metab. **2** (1988) 591−617.

[3] Baroni, C. D., L. Manente, V. Maccallini et al.: Primary malignant tumors of the thyroid gland. Histology, age and sex distribution and pathologic correlations in 139 cases. Tumori **69** (1983) 205−213.

[4] Blum, C. J., C. Lafont, M. Ducasse et al.: Thyroid function tests in aging and their relation to associated nonthyroidal disease. J. Endocrinol. Invest. **12** (1989) 307−312.

[5] Blumenthal, H. T., I. B. Perlstein: The aging thyroid. I. A description of lesions and an analysis of their age and sex distribution. J. Am. Geriatr. Soc. **35** (1987) 843−854.

[6] Brik, H., A. Shainberg: Thyroxine induced transitions of red towards white muscle in cultured heart cells. Basic Res. Cardiol. **85** (1990) 237−246.

[7] Brun, R., M. Jenny, J. P. Junod: Hyperthyroidism in older patients. Schweiz. Med. Wochenschr. **108** (1978) 1504−1510.

[8] Butler, J. S., Jr., L. W. Brady, B. E. Amendola: Lymphoma of the thyroid. Report of five cases and review. Am. J. Clin. Oncol. **13** (1990) 64−69.

[9] Campos-Pastor, M. M., M. Munoz-Torres, F. Escobar-Jimenez et al.: Bone mass in females with different thyroid disorders: influence of menopausal status. Bone Miner. **21** (1993) 1−8.

[10] Casiglia, E., O. Maschio, P. Spolaore et al.: Atrial fibrillation in a cohort of the elderly: etiopathogenetic role of occult hyperthyroidism and diagnostic and therapeutic considerations. Result of the CASTEL (Cardiovascular Study in the Elderly). Cardiologia **36** (1991) 685−691.

[11] Cobler, J. L., M. E. Williams, P. Greenland: Thyrotoxicosis in institutionalized elderly patients with atrial fibrillation. Arch. Intern. Med. **144** (1984) 1758−1760.

[12] Compagno, J., J. E. Oertel: Malignant lymphoma and other lymphoproliferative disorders of the thyroid gland. A clinicopathologic study of 245 cases. Am. J. Clin. Pathol. **74** (1980) 1−11.

[13] Danforth, E., A. G. Burger: The impact of nutrition on thyroid hormone physiology and action. Ann. Rev. Nutr. **9** (1989) 201−227.

[14] Davis, P. J., F. B. Davis: Hyperthyroidism in patients over the age of 60 years. Clinical features in 85 patients. Medicine (Baltimore) **53** (1974) 161−181.

[15] de Carvalho-Filho, E. T., V. L. Dias, M. C. Fernandes et al.: Cardiac manifestations of hyperthyroidism in the elderly. Arg. Bras. Cardiol. **56** (1991) 31−37.

[16] Demeester-Mirkine, N., M. Kutnowski, B. Futeral et al.: Thyroid status in elderly sick patients. J. Endocrinol. Invest. **4** (1981) 41−44.

[17] Denham, M. J., E. J. Wills: A clinico-pathological survey of thyroid glands in old age. Gerontology **26** (1980) 160−166.

[18] Diamond, T., J. Vine, R. Smart et al.: Thyrotoxic bone disease in women: a potentially reversible disorder. Ann. Intern. Med. **120** (1994) 8−11.

[19] Dillman, W. H.: Biochemical basis of thyroid hormone action in the heart. Am. J. Med. **88** (1990) 626−630.

[20] Doniach, D., G. F. Bottazzo, R. C. Russell: Goitrous autoimmune thyroiditis (Hashimoto's disease). Clin. Endocrinol. Metab. **8** (1979) 63−80.

[21] Eulry, F., B. Bauduceau, D. Lechevalier et al.: Bone density in differentiated cancer of the thyroid gland treated by hormone-suppressive therapy. Study based on 51 cases. Rev. Rhum. Mal. Osteoartic. **59** (1992) 247−252.

[22] Featherstone, H. J., D. K. Stewart: Angina in thyrotoxicosis. Thyroid-related coronary artery spasm. Arch. Intern. Med. **143** (1983) 554−555.

[23] Felicetta, J. V.: The thyroid and aging. In: Jr. R. Sowers, J. V. Felicetta (eds.): The endocrinology of aging, pp. 15−39. Raven Press, New York 1988.

[24] Florkowski, C. M., B. E. Brownlie, J. R. Elliot et al.: Bone mineral density in patients receiving suppressive doses of thyroxine for thyroid carcinoma. N. Z. Med. J. **106** (1993) 443−444.

[25] Foldes, J., G. Tarjan, M. Szathmari et al.: Bone mineral density in patients with endogenous subclinical hyperthyroidism: is this thyroid status a risk factor for osteoporosis? Clin. Endocrinol. (Oxf.) 39 (1993) 521−527.

[26] Franklyn, J. A., J. Betteridge, J. Daykin et al.: Long-term thyroxine treatment and bone mineral density. Lancet 340 (1992) 9−13.

[27] Gaffney, G. W., R. I. Gregerman, N. W. Shok: Relationship of age to the thyroidal accumulation, renal excretion and distribution of radioiodide in euthyroid subjects. J. Clin. Endocrinol. Metab. 22 (1962) 784−794.

[28] Gerber, D.: Thyroid weights and iodized salt prophylaxis: a comparative study from autopsy material from the Institute of Pathology, University of Zurich. Schweiz. Med. Wochenschr. 110 (1980) 2010−2017.

[29] Goichot, B., J. L. Schlienger, F. Grunenberger et al.: Thyroid hormone status and nutrient intake in the free-living elderly. Interest of reverse triiodothyronine assessment. Eur. J. Endocrinol. 130 (1994) 244−252.

[30] Grant, D. J., M. E. McMurdo, P. A. Mole et al.: Suppressed TSH levels secondary to thyroxine replacement therapy are not associated with osteoporosis. Clin. Endocrinol. (Oxf.) 39 (1993) 529−533.

[31] Gregerman, R. I., G. W. Gaffney, N. W. Shok: Thyroxine turnover in euthyroid man with special reference to changes in age. J. Clin. Invest. 41 (1962) 2065−2074.

[32] Hansen, J. M:, L. Skovsted, K. Siersbaek-Nielsen: Age dependent changes in iodine metabolism and thyroid function. Acta Endocrinol. (Copenh.) 79 (1975) 60−65.

[33] Harman, S. M., R. E. Wehmann, M. R. Blackman: Pituitary-thyroid hormone economy in healthy aging men: basal indices of thyroid function and thyrotropin responses to constant infusions of thyrotropin releasing hormone. J. Clin. Endocrinol. Metab. 58 (1984) 320−326.

[34] Hegedus, L., H. Perrild, L. R. Poulsen et al.: The determination of thyroid volume by ultrasound and its relationship to body weight, age, and sex in normal subjects. J. Clin. Endocrinol. Metab. 56 (1983) 260−263.

[35] Heimann, R.: Primary malignant lymphomas of the thyroid. A brief review. Acta Otorhinolaryngol. Belg. 41 (1987) 727−735.

[36] Herrmann, J.: Prevalence of hypothyroidism in the elderly in Germany. A pilot study. J. Endocrinol. Invest. 4 (1981) 327−330.

[37] Hershman, J. M., A. E. Pekary, L. Berg et al.: Serum thyrotropin and thyroid hormone levels in elderly and middle-aged euthyroid persons. J. Am. Geriatr. Soc. 41 (1993) 823−828.

[38] Hesch, R. D., J. Gatz, H. Juppner et al.: TBG-dependency of age related variations of thyroxine and triiodothyronine. Horm. Metab. Res. 9 (1977) 141−146.

[39] Hintze, G., J. Windeler, J. Baumert et al.: Thyroid volume and goiter prevalence in the elderly as determined by ultrasound and their relationships to laboratory indices. Acta Endocrinol. (Copenh.) 124 (1991) 12−18.

[40] Hrafnkelsson, J., O. Stal, S. Enestrom et al.: Cellular DNA pattern, S-phase frequency and survival in papillary thyroid cancer. Acta Oncol. 27 (1988) 329−333.

[41] Joensuu, H., P. Klemi, E. Eerola et al.: Influence of cellular DNA content on survival in differentiated thyroid cancer. Cancer 58 (1986) 2462−2467.

[42] Kabadi, U. M., P. M. Rosman: Thyroid hormone indices in adult healthy subjects: no influence of aging. J. Am. Geriatr. Soc. 36 (1988) 312−316.

[43] Koike, A., T. Naruse: Incidence of thyroid cancer in Japan. Semin. Surg. Oncol. 7 (1991) 107−111.

[44] Kung, A. W., T. Lorentz, S. C. Tam: Thyroxine suppressive therapy decreases bone mineral density in post-menopausal women. Clin. Endocrinol. (Oxf.) 39 (1993) 535−540.

[45] Kurashima, C., K. Hirokawa: Focal lymphocytic infiltration in thyroids of elderly people. Histopathological and immunohistochemical studies. Surv. Synth. Pathol. Res. **4** (1985) 457−466.

[46] Ladenson, P. W.: Thyrotoxicosis and the heart: Something old something new. J. Clin. Endocrinol. Metab. **77** (1993) 332−333.

[47] Laurberg, P., K. M. Pedersen, H. Vestergaard et al.: High incidence of multinodular toxic goitre in the elderly population in a low iodine intake area vs. high incidence of Graves' disease in the young in a high iodine intake area: comparative surveys of thyrotoxicosis epidemiology in East-Jutland Denmark and Iceland. J. Intern. Med. **229** (1991) 415−420.

[48] Lehmke, J., U. Bogner, D. Felsenberg et al.: Determination of bone mineral density by quantitative computed tomography and single photon absorptiometry in subclinical hyperthyroidism: a risk of early osteopaenia in post-menopausal women. Clin. Endocrinol. (Oxf.) **36** (1992) 511−517.

[49] Machill, K., G. H. Scholz: Dependence of hemodynamic changes in hyperthyroidism on age of patients and etiology of hyperthyroidism. In: L. E. Braverman, O. Eber, W. Langsteger (eds.): Heart and thyroid, pp. 76−83. Blackwell-MZV, Graz 1994.

[50] Mariotti, S., G. Barbesino, P. Caturegli et al.: Complex alteration of thyroid function in healthy centenarians. J. Clin. Endocrinol. Metab. **77** (1993) 1130−1134.

[51] Mariotti, S., P. Sansoni, G. Barbesino et al.: Thyroid and other organ-specific autoantibodies in healthy centenarians. Lancet **339** (1992) 1506−1508.

[52] Melmed, S., Hershman, J. M.: The thyroid and aging. In: S. G. Korenman (ed.): Endocrine aspects of aging, pp. 33−53. Elsevier Biomedical, New York 1982.

[53] Moliterno, D., C. R. DeBold, R. M. Robertson: Case report: Coronary vasospasm − relation to the hyperthyroid state. Am. J. Med. Sci. **304** (1992) 38−42.

[54] Mortensen, J. D., L. B. Woolner, W. A. Bennett: Gross and microscopic findings in clinically normal thyroid glands. In: Transactions of the American Goiter Association, pp. 1270−1280. Charles C. Thomas, 1956.

[55] Ohishi, T., M. Takahashi, K. Kushida et al.: Quantitative analyses of urinary pyridinoline and deoxypyridinoline excretion in patients with hyperthyroidism. Endocr. Res. **18** (1992) 281−290.

[56] Okayasu, I., S. Hatakeyama, Y. Tanaka et al.: Is focal chronic autoimmune thyroiditis an age-related disease? Differences in incidence and severity between Japanese and British J. Pathol. **163** (1991) 257−264.

[57] Parle, J. V., J. A. Franklyn, K. W. Cross et al.: Prevalence and follow-up of abnormal thyrotrophin (TSH) concentrations in the elderly in the United Kingdom. Clin. Endocrinol. (Oxf.) **34** (1991) 77−83.

[58] Perros, P., A. L. Crombie, J. N. Matthews et al.: Age and gender influence the severity of thyroid-associated ophthalmopathy: a study of 101 patients attending a combined thyroid-eye clinic. Clin. Endocrinol. (Oxf.) **38** (1993) 367−372.

[59] Pioli, G., M. Pedrazzoni, E. Palummeri et al.: Longitudinal study of bone loss after thyroidectomy and suppressive thyroxine therapy in premenopausal women. Acta Endocrinol. (Copenh.) **126** (1992) 238−242.

[60] Raue, F., M. Späth-Schröder, J. Winter et al.: Register für das medulläre Schilddrüsenkarzinom in der Bundesrepublik Deutschland. Med. Klin. **85** (1990) 113−116.

[61] Reeve, T. S., L. Delbridge, P. Crummer: Total thyroidectomy in the management of differentiated thyroid cancer: a review of 258 cases. Aust. N. Z. J. Surg. **56** (1986) 829−833.

[62] Riddell, D. A., H. B. Lampe, H. Cramer et al.: Medullary thyroid carcinoma: prognostic factors. J. Otolaryngol. **22** (1993) 180−183.

[63] Robuschi, G., M. Safran, L. E. Braverman et al.: Hypothyroidism in the elderly. Endocr. Rev. **8** (1987) 142−153.

[64] Ronnov-Jessen, V., C. Kirkegaard: Hyperthyroidism − a disease of old age? Br. Med. J. 1 (1973) 41−43.

[65] Rosenthal, M. J., W. C. Hunt, P. J. Garry et al.: Thyroid failure in the elderly. Microsomal antibodies as discriminant for therapy. JAMA 258 (1987) 209−213.

[66] Ross, D. S.: Bone density is not reduced during the short-term administration of levothyroxine to postmenopausal women with subclinical hypothyroidism: a randomized, prospective study. Am. J. Med. 95 (1993) 385−388.

[67] Rossmanith, W. G., A. Szilagyi, W. A. Scherbaum: Episodic thyrotropin (TSH) and prolactin (PRL) secretion during aging in postmenopausal women. Horm. metab. Res. 24 (1992) 185−190.

[68] Roti, E., E. Gardini, R. Minelli et al.: Prevalence of anti-thyroid peroxidase antibodies in serum in the elderly: comparison with other tests for anti-thyroid antibodies. Clin. Chem. 38 (1992) 88−92.

[69] Sawin, C. T., S. T. Bigos, S. Land et al.: The aging thyroid. Relationship between elevated serum thyrotropin level and thyroid antibodies in elderly patients. Am. J. Med. 79 (1985) 591−595.

[70] Sawin, C. T., W. P. Castelli, J. M. Hershman et al.: The aging thyroid. Thyroid deficiency in the Framingham Study. Arch. Intern. Med. 145 (1985) 1386−1388.

[71] Sawin, C. T., D. Chopra, F. Azizi et al.: The aging thyroid. Increased prevalence of elevated serum thyrotropin levels in the elderly. JAMA 242 (1979) 247−250.

[72] Schaaf, L., M. Greschner, R. Paschke et al.: Thyrotoxic crisis in Graves' disease: indication for immediate surgery. Klin. Wochenschr. 68 (1990) 1037−1041.

[73] Scherbaum, W. A., G. Stöckle, J. Wichmann et al.: Immunological and clinical characterization of patients with untreated euthyroid and hypothyroid autoimmune thyroiditis. Antibody spectrum, response to TRH and clinical study. Acta Endocrinol. (Copenh.) 100 (1982) 373−381.

[74] Simons, R. J., J. M. Simon, L. M. Demers et al.: Thyroid dysfunction in elderly hospitalized patients. Effect of age and severity of illness. Arch. Intern. Med. 150 (1990) 1249−1253.

[75] Sisson, J. C.: Medical treatment of benign and malignant thyroid tumors. Endocrinol. Metab. Clin. North. Am. 18 (1989) 359−387.

[76] Slag, M. F., J. E. Morley, M. K. Elson et al.: Hypothyroxinemia in critically ill patients as a predictor of high mortality. JAMA 245 (1981) 43−45.

[77] Small, D., W. Gibbons, R. D. Levy: Exertional dyspnea and ventilation in hyperthyroidism. Chest 101 (1992) 1268−1273.

[78] Snyder, P. J., R. D. Utiger: Response to thyrotropin releasing hormone (TRH) in normal man. J. Clin. Endocrinol. Metab. 34 (1972) 380−385.

[79] Stockigt, J. R.: Prescribing for the elderly. Thyroid disease. Med. J. Aust. 158 (1994) 770−774.

[80] Sugino, K., Y. Kure, O. Ozaki et al.: Does L-thyroxine administration in a dose to suppress TSH secretion induce metabolic bone disturbance in patients with thyroid carcinoma?. Nippon. Geka. Gakkai. Zasshi. 93 (1992) 753−756.

[81] Tak, P. P., J. Hermans, A. Haak: Symptomatology of Graves' disease and Plummer's disease in relation to age and thyroid hormone level. Neth. J. Med. 42 (1993) 157−162.

[82] Tibaldi, J. M., U. S. Barzel, J. Albin et al.: Thyrotoxicosis in the very old. Am. J. Med. 81 (1986) 619−622.

[83] Tunbridge, W. M., D. C. Evered, R. Hall et al.: The spectrum of thyroid disease in a community: the Whickham survey. Clin. Endocrinol. (Oxf.) 7 (1977) 481−493.

[84] Urban, R. J., J. D. Veldhuis: Hypothalamo-pituitary concomitants of aging. In: J. R. Sowers, J. V. Felicetta (eds.): The endocrinology of aging, pp. 74−81. Raven Press, New York 1988.

[85] van Coevorden, A., E. Laurent, C. Decoster et al.: Decreased basal and stimulated thyrotropin secretion in healthy elderly men. J. Clin. Endocrinol. Metab. 69 (1989) 177−185.

[86] Wainstein, E., A. Castillo, G. Pineda: Problems in the diagnosis of thyroid dysfunction of the elderly adult. Rev. Med. Chil. **118** (1990) 405–413.
[87] Wenzel, K. W., W. R. Horn: Triiodothyronine (T3) and thyroxine (T4) kinetics in aged men. In: J. Robbins et al. (eds.): Thyroid research, pp. 270–273. Excerpta Medica, Amsterdam 1976.

The influence of aging on thyroxine 5'-deiodinating activity in cultivated adipocyte precursors

Ch.-F. Wolf, E. Kubbutat, B. Wagner, L. Duntas, J. Wieberneit, F. S. Keck

Introduction

The main source of intracellular and circulating 3,5,3'-Triiodothyronine (T_3) in humans is the extrathyroidal phenolic 5'deiodination (5'D) of Thyroxine (T_4). Reduced serum levels of T_3, normal or reduced serum levels of TSH and alterations in 5'Deiodinating Activity have been described both as "euthyroid sick syndrome" and as an aspect of aging [4, 11]. We have studied the possible influence of aging on 5'D in cultured human adipocyte precursors. Aging was determined as the mere passing of time, as the quantity of cell proliferation and as the period of recovery following traumatic events. The interval of time following "cell splitting" was chosen as a parameter of aging because 5'D is augmented directly following this traumatic situation.

In addition to the properties of aging, it is reasonable to feature 5'D in adipose tissue for two further physiological aspects: i. interactions between thyroid hormones and lipid metabolism have numerous physiological aspects; ii. the distribution of total T_3 in human covers by 76% the "slow pool" (which is represented in white adipose tissue [3], muscle, skin and gut) by 19% the "fast pool" (e. g. liver, kidney; both type I 5'D) and by 5% the plasma [3]. The 5'D in human adipose tissue is of type II [9, 13]. Intracellular (5'D) has been demonstrated to depend upon a variety of metabolic conditions, e. g. thyroid state [6, 8], catecholamine status [12] and glucose metabolism [5]. Employing the tool of cell cultivation we have been able to keep each of these factors constant. By excluding the metabolic influences we have isolated the factor "aging" in the experimental design.

Methods

Cell cultivation was performed as previously described [13], in short: Human adipocyte precursors were isolated by collagenous digestion from truncal subcutaneous adipose tissue. Separated cells were cultured in Ham's F-12/DMEM (50/50; v/v) and 10% FCS. Cultivation medium was continuously supplemented. Cells were kept at 37 °C (CO_2: 5%). Confluent culture dishes were either harvested by "cell-scraping" for the determination of 5'deiodinating activity or splittet for further cell cultivation. "Cell splitting" employed digestion with Trypsin (2 g/dl in PBS) for two minutes followed by cell cultivation in new culture dishes. 5'deiodinating activity was determined in isolated microsomes obtained by differential centrifugation. Microsomal protein (400 µg) was incubated together with T_4 (1 and 5 µM) at 37 °C over 12 hours and newly generated T_3 was determined radio-immunologically. 5'deiodinating activity was calculated as T_3/h · mg (prot.). The validity of the method was checked by measurement of the release of radio-labelled iodine from ^{125}J 5'-labelled-T_4 in incubation, as well as by the study of rT_3-decomposition in incubation. 5'D in cells deriving from the same donor (♂, 46 y.) was monitored over four months. The cell proliferation number (P; calculated cell divisions), the duration of cell cultivation (C; days), and the time period after cell splitting (S) were considered as possible factors of influence on 5'deiodinating activity. Statistical analysis was done by Pearson's simple correlation coefficient (r_S) and by calculating first-order and second-order partial correlations (r_P) keeping constant (const.) one or two of the possibly 5'D influencing factors (F) under consideration.

Results

The intracellular 5'deiodinating activity in adipocyte precursors declined over the observation period. This decrease can be expressed in days of cell cultivation (d; Fig. 1), or in observed cell proliferation (cell reproduction: "n"; Fig. 1). In constrast, an increase in 5'deiodinating activity was observed as related to the interval of time (d) passing after any cell splitting performed (Fig. 2).

The statistical analysis of the factors influencing 5'D in cell cultivation yielded the identification of the "period of recovery after the event of cell splitting"

Table 1   Pearson's partial correlations coefficient $r_{(p)}$ by calculating first-order and second-order correlations keeping constant (const.) one or two of the possibly 5'D influencing factors (F) under consideration. The calculated probabilities (p) for the error of the first kind demonstrate the interval of cultivation as the predominant factor influencing 5'deiodinating activity.

F1	5'D	5'D	5'D	5'D	5'D	5'D	5'D	5'D
F2	P	P	C	S	C	S	S	C
const.	C	S	P	P	S	C	C, P	P, S
r	−0.47	−0.25	−0.31	0.40	−0.34	0.561	0.37	−0.06
p	n. s.	n. s.	n. s.	n. s.	n. s.	0.05	n. s.	n. s.

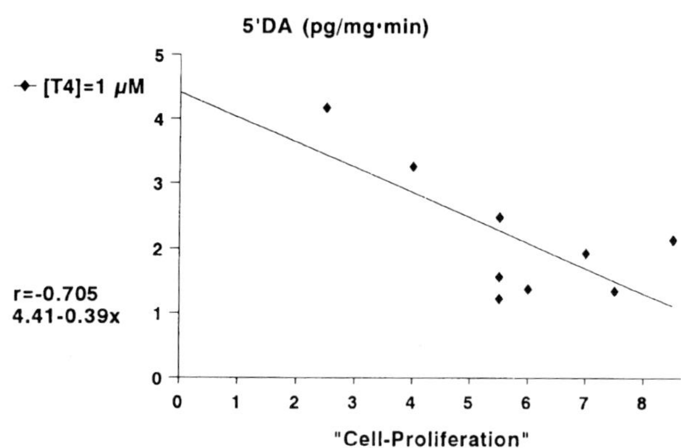

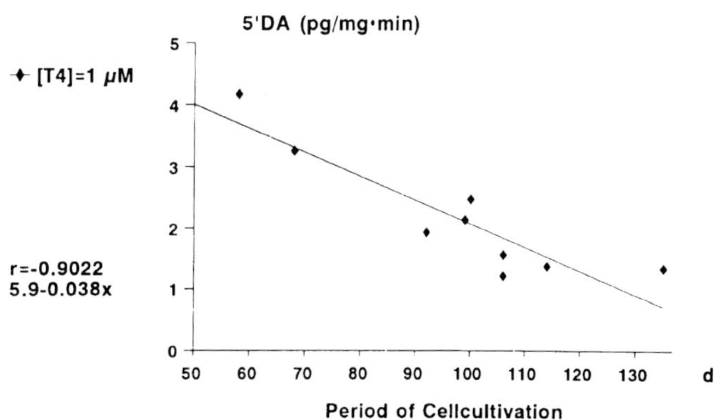

Fig. 1 T_4 to T_3 5'Deiodinating Activity (pg/mg · min) expressed as decrease of the enzymatic activity over the cultivation period and as decrease of the enzymatic activity over the cell proliferation (2^a).

factor as the strongest component regulating 5'deiodinating activity (Table 1, Fig. 2). However, keeping the "cell proliferation" factor (C) constant, the significance of the factor P vanishes.

Discussion and conclusion

Our data demonstrate the decrease of 5'deiodinating activity by approximately 50% over a cell cultivation period of 4 months. The decrease can be presented

T4 - 5'DEIODINATION

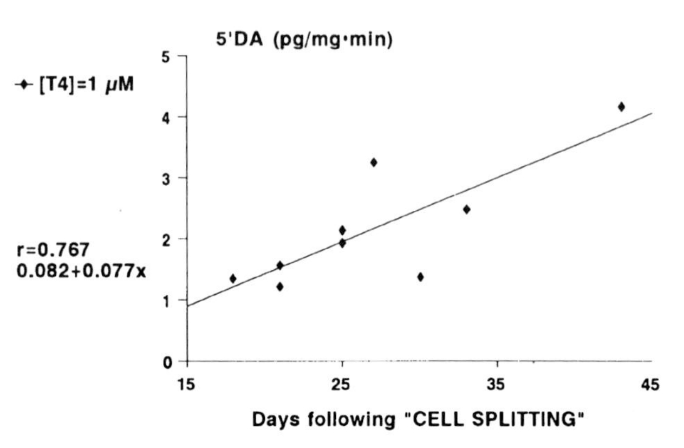

- Period of Cellcultivation -
- Days following "Cell Splitting" -

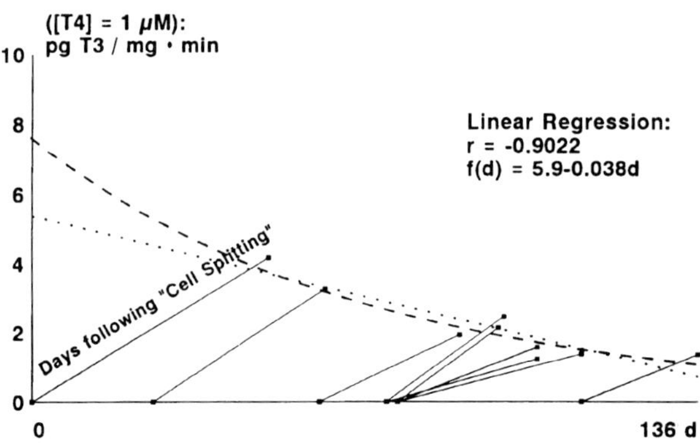

Fig. 2 T_4 to T_3 5'deiodinating activity (pg/mg · min) expressed as increase of the enzymatic activity as detected after "cell splitting".

as a function of both the period of cell cultivation and the estimated cell proliferation. Between these two influencing factors, we have identified the period of cell cultivation as the major determinant for 5'deiodinating activity by Pearson's simple correlation coefficient (r_S) and Pearson's partial correlations (r_P). Since the factor "C" obviously does disturb the correlation of 5'D and P, an additional 5'deiodinating activity reducing effect by cell proliferation cannot be excluded.

Our finding of the increase of 5'deiodinating activity as related to the interval of time following the event of "cell-splitting" contradicts the assumed hypothesis of a 5'D-depressing effect by cultivation media. However, as demonstrated in Fig. 2, the period of recovery of 5'D following the event of "cell-splitting" fundamentally determines the detected increasing activities of 5'D in the harvested cells.

A potential to generate T_3 out of T_4 was observed in our cultured cells four months after isolation out of human fat pads. Regarding other essential enzymic systems, in adipocyte precursors such general enzymic activity is not found. The ability to differentiate to adipocytes under physiological stimuli vanishes within the first 24 hours after isolation from adipose tissue pads [7]. Although lipid metabolism in cultured adipocyte precursors appears to be altered after a few days of cells cultivation, studies regarding T_4-metabolism in cultured mortal cells do report detectable enzymatic activities for longer periods of cell cultivation [2, 10].

The discrepancy between the development of the specific enzymic activities during cell cultivation restrains the option to employ cell cultivating systems as a model for "in vivo aging". However, the observed decrease in 5'D over the cultivation period may feature at least the effects of "in-vitro aging" and may furthermore give an additional aspect for the handling of data deriving from studies in mortal cells regarding 5'D.

In-vivo alterations of 5'deiodinating activity as related to aging have been described for type I and type II deiodination in liver, thyroid and pituitary [4]. Data regarding the alteration of the endocrinologically active enzyme "aromatase" give evidence that at least some enzymic activities in the human adipose tissue are age-related in-vivo [1]. Reflecting upon our data, we can conclude that the reduction of 5'deiodinating activity as related to "in-vitro aging" in cultured human adipocyte precursors, is primarily a function of the periods of recovery following to the traumatic events of cell splitting. The decrease of 5'deiodinating activity as demonstrated over the observed period of cell cultivation therefore results from the frequency of exogenous injury.

References

[1] Cleland, H. W., C. R. Mendelson, E. R. Simpson: Effects of aging and obesity on aromatase activity of human adipose cells. J. Clin. Endocrinol. Metab. **60** (1985) 174−177.

[2] Courtin, F., F. Chantoux, J. Francon: Thyroid hormone metabolism in neuron-enriched primary cultures of fetal rat brain cells. Mol. Cell. Endocr. **58** (1988) 73−84.

[3] Di Stefano III, J. J.: Modelling approaches and models of the distribution and disposal of thyroid hormones: In: G. Hennemann (Hrsg.): Thyroid hormone metabolism, S. 39−76. Marcel Dekker INC, New York 1986.

[4] Donda, A., T. Lemarchand-Beraud: Aging alters the activity of 5'-deiodinase in the adenohypophysis, thyroid gland, and liver of the male rat. Endocrinol. **124** (1989) 1305−1309.

[5] Grau, R., F. S. Keck et al.: The influence of glucose and insulin infusion on in vitro T4 monodeiodination in rat liver microsomes. Horm. Metab. Res. **14** (1984) 62−65.

[6] Grussendorf, M., M. Hüfner: Induction of the thyroxine (T4) to triiodothyronine (T3) converting enzyme in rat liver by thyroid hormones and analogs. Clin. Chim. Acta **80** (1977) 61−66.

[7] Hauner, H., G. Entenmann et al.: Differentiation of human adipocyte precursors in a chemically defined medium. J. Clin. Invest. **84** (1989) 1663−1667.

[8] Keck, F. S., Ch.-F. Wolf, E. F. Pfeiffer: The influence of circulating thyroxine serum concentration on hepatic thyroxine deiodination activity in rats. Exp. Clin. Endocrinol. **96** (1990) 269−279.

[9] Nauman, A., J. Nauman et al.: Thyroxine 5'-deiodinase in human adipose tissue. In: P. Björntorp, S. Rössner (Hrsg.): Obesity in Europe 88, S. 177−183. John Libbey, London−Paris 1988.

[10] Safran, M., J. L. Leonard: Comparison of the physicochemical properties of type I and type II iodothyronine 5'-deiodinase. J. Biol. Chem. **266** (1991) 3233−3238.

[11] Schroffner, W. G.: The aging thyroid in health and disease. Geriatrics **42** (1987) 41−43, 48.

[12] Wolf, Ch.-F., F. S. Keck et al.: In vivo modulation of 5'deiodinating activity in rat liver microsomes. J. Gen. Comparat. Endocrinol. **74** (1989) 287−288.

[13] Wolf, Ch.-F., J. Wieberneit et al: Deiodination of thyroxine and reverse triiodothyronine in cells of human adipose tissue. In: H. F. Deckart, E. Strehlau (Hrsg.): New Aspects in Thyroid Disease, S. 96−102. Walter de Gruyter, Berlin−New York 1992.

Degradation of intravenously administered thyrotropin-releasing hormone in the elderly

L. Duntas, B. M. Grab, Ch.-F. Wolf, U. Loos, F. S. Keck

Introduction

The enzymatic degradation of thyrotropin-releasing hormone (TRH) must be taken into consideration when studying the function and/or the duration of TRH action. In adult humans, the duration of TRH actions is dependent upon regulation by the degradation system. The main regulators of enzymatic inactivation of TRH are the thyroid hormones [1]. The deamidization of TRH is catalyzed by a post-proline cleaving enzyme and the hydrolysis of TRH at the pyroGlu-His bond by a pyroglutamate aminopeptidase [2]. No studies have been performed on the age-related rate of TRH degradation in plasma. The aims of this study were to derive information on the metabolic rate of TRH in the elderly and to obtain basic kinetic data on TRH using a single-compartment model in healthy elderly men as compared to young adults.

Methods

Subjects and study protocol

Nine euthyroid men aged 65−71 years (mean 69 years) and six control subjects aged 27−44 years (mean 36 years) participated in this study. Two patients had a macrocytic (Hb: 10.9 and 11.8 g/dl; MCV: 113 and 100 fl and MCH: 35.4 and 35.7 pg respectively) and one a microcytic anemia (Hb: 12.1; MCV: 80 fl and MCH: 30.2 pg). A standard TRH-test (Antepan^R 200 µg, Henning-Berlin GmbH) was performed intravenously in all subjects. Blood samples for determination of serum TSH and plasma TRH concentrations were collected before and at 2, 5, 10, 20, 30 and 60 minutes after TRH injection. Plasma TRH was determined after extraction by a sensitive RIA as previously reported [2]. The intra-assay and inter-assay coefficients of variation (CV) were calculated at 4.8% and 4% respectively. The sensitivity was 1 pg (3 fmol/tube). The normal range for blood TRH was fixed at 20−80 fmol/ml. Serum concentrations of TSH were measured by immunoluminometric assay (LUMItest-TSH, Henning-Berlin GmbH) with intra-assay CV of 5.2%.

Statistics

The half-life $(t_{1/2})$ of TRH was calculated from the log-transformation of its plasma concentration. The relationship between time and plasma concentration was described by linear regression. As the half-life is the time taken for a 50% reduction in concentration, it can be calculated by dividing 0.693 (i. e. ln 2) by the slope of the regression line. The procedures used and their accuracy have been detailed previously [3].

Results

Plasma concentrations after administering TRH, and half-lives of TRH obtained from bolus injection in the control group and in the elderly, are shown in Fig. 1 and 2. No significant alterations were observed in C_{max} (13487 $\pm$ 267 vs. 16824 $\pm$ 3951 fmol/ml) or in t_{max} of TRH (2 min) between the elderly and the control group. In contrast, patients with anemia showed a prolonged $t_{1/2}$ (8.7 min) and a larger C_{max} (38252 $\pm$ 10671 fmol/ml) after injection of TRH (Fig. 3). TSH serum concentrations during the basal period and 30 min after TRH administration were not significantly different between groups. The basal and reactive after TRH injection TSH values were all in normal range (from 1.1 $\pm$ 0.3 (SD) to 11.3 $\pm$ 1.8 μU/ml, and from 0.9 $\pm$ 0.1 to 8.5 $\pm$ 1.4 μU/ml, respectively). However, a reduced δ-TSH was observed in the elderly group, 10.2 vs. 7.6 μU/ml, as compared with the controls.

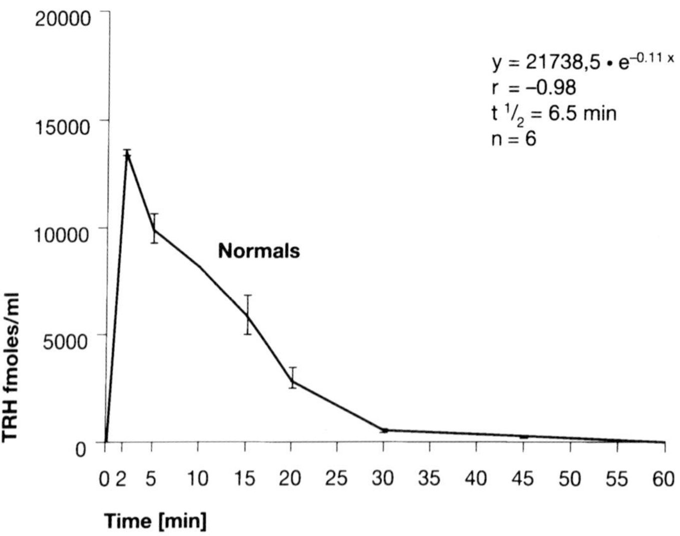

Fig. 1 Kinetics of plasma TRH concentrations after TRH administration in six normal young adult subjects.

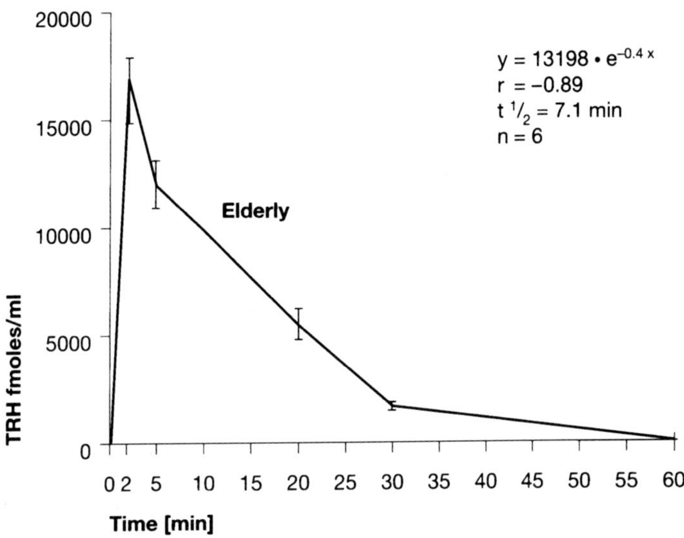

Fig. 2 Kinetics of plasma TRH concentrations after TRH administration in the elderly.

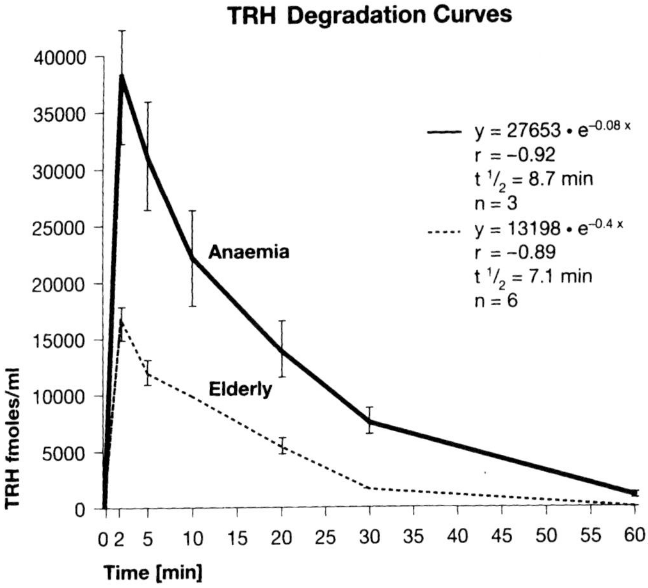

Fig. 3 Kinetics of plasma TRH concentrations after TRH administration in six euthyroid normal elderly men and in three elderly men with anemia.

Discussion

These results demonstrate that the half-life of exogenous TRH given as a bolus injection in older subjects is only slightly prolonged as compared to young adults. In contrast, patients with anemia had markedly prolonged half-lives. This could not be attributed to an effect of thyroid hormones, (e. g. of latent hypothyroidism) because the thyroid hormones and TSH serum concentrations were normal. These findings might be explained as a consequence of the decreased erythrocyte-, plasma- and enzymatic-concentration in the anemic patients. Additionally, we cannot exclude an altered clearance in these patients, since TRH decline is a function of compartmental flux, plasma degradation and renal clearance.

The elderly subjects demonstrated no significant changes in either magnitude or timing of TSH responses to TRH. The differences observed in elderly patients with anemia showed no correlation to the TRH induced TSH increase, suggesting that extravascular TRH degradation and/or a possible age-related diminution in pituitary TRH binding sites may be of some importance in TSH regulation.

References

[1] Bauer, K: Regulation of degradation of thyrotropin-releasing hormone by thyroid hormones. Nature **259** (1976) 591−593.
[2] Bauer, K., P. Nowak, H. Kleinkauf: Specificity of a serum peptidase hydrolyzing thyroliberin at the pyroglutamyl-histidine bond. Eur. J. Biochem. **178** (1981) 173−176.
[3] Duntas, L., F. S. Keck, D. Grouselle, J. Rosenthal et al.: Thyrotropin-releasing hormone: further extraction studies and analysis by fast protein liquid chromatography and radioimmunoassay. J. Endocrinol. Invest. **14** (1991) 173−179.

Pituitary-adrenocortical dysfunctions in the elderly

H. L. Fehm, Ch. Dodt, E. Späth-Schwalbe, W. Kern, J. Born

Introduction

The prominent role of hormones in the control of normal growth and development has been acknowledged for many years. The corresponding idea of hormones playing a similar role in the control of normal processes of senescence, has been considered only recently [13]. Promotion of these concepts was provided by the "glucocorticoid cascade hypothesis" put forth by Sapolsky et al. 1986 [16]. This hypothesis, based on experimental work in rats [15, 17], proposes that aging results from deterioration of neuroendocrine functions. These authors observed elevated basal and peak corticosterone levels in response to stressful stimuli as well as prolonged adrenal secretion in old rats as compared with young controls. Along with these humoral changes, old animals exhibited neuronal damage in the hippocampus, which was attributed to toxic effects of the elevated corticosterone levels. These lesions, in turn, are thought to impair an inhibitory influence of hippocampal neurons on the hypophysial secretory activity, thus priming a vicious cycle with even further prolonged activity of the pituitary-adrenal system under stess conditions [12].

All studies mentioned so far have utilized rats. While most of the features of Sapolsky's hypothesis appear to be potentially operable in the human brain and endocrine system, the existing data argue against the syndrome of glucocorticoid hypersecretion as a normative part of human aging [3, 11].

These inconsistencies led us to re-evaluate the functions of the **brain-pituitary-adrenocortical (BPA) system** in mentally and physically healthy aged human subjects. We examined (i) the effect of old age on the response of the BPA system to stimulation using different secretagogues, and (ii) the effect of age on basal cortisol secretion, especially on nadir cortisol levels. (iii) Evidence will be provided that peptide hormones of the BPA system (ACTH and vasopressin) influence CNS functions in the elderly in an age-specific manner.

Responsiveness of the BPA system

In a pilot experiment we studied the response of plasma cortisol to simultaneous intravenous administration of hCRH (50 µg) and lysin-vasopressin (0.5

I. U.). A group of 12 healthy subjects older than 70 years was compared with subjects 20−30 years of age. Basal cortisol levels were higher in the elderly and the typical decline during the rest-period before administration of the stimulus (at 10.00 h) was attenuated (Fig. 1). In spite of the elevated starting levels which usually blunt the response, the CRH/LVP induced increase was similar in both groups. Also in both groups cortisol levels returned to initial levels with comparable velocity. Thus cortisol levels in the aged exceeded those of young controls throughout the observation period. These results are in some aspects similar to those observed by Sapolsky in old rats. However, other investigators using human or ovine CRH but not VP as stimulus found unchanged or even blunted responses in old subjects [9, 14, 18, 21].

To exclude the possibility that an enhanced response to stimulation in the elderly occurs only with VP and not with CRH we studied the ACTH and cortisol responses to stimulation with either 100 µg hCRH plus 0.5 I. U. LVP or

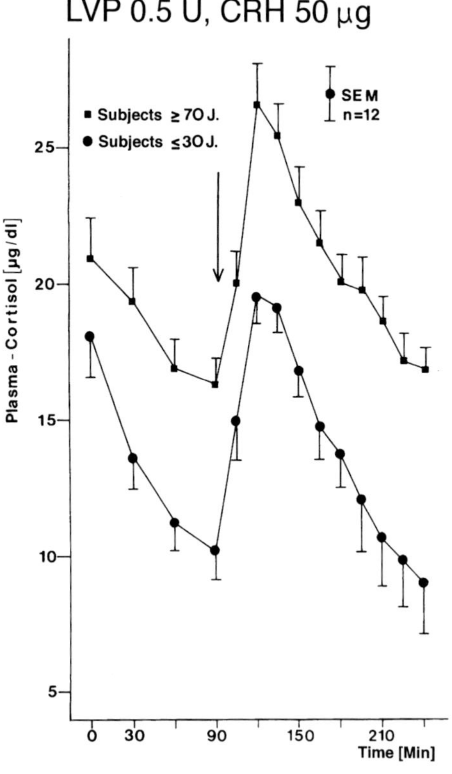

Fig. 1   Plasma cortisol response to stimulation with hCRH + LVP in 12 healthy subjects older than 70 yrs and in young controls (26−30 yrs). LVP, lysin-vasopressin; hCRH, human corticotropin releasing hormone.

hCRH alone in a group of 10 healthy old subjects (78−92 years). All tests were performed in the afternoon, starting at 16.00 h. During the 60 minute baseline period there were no differences in plasma ACTH and cortisol levels as compared with a group of young subjects (21−27 years old). However, after stimulation with either hCRH/LVP or hCRH alone, the elderly exhibited strikingly higher plasma ACTH and cortisol levels (Fig. 2). Especially plasma ACTH levels were in most of the aged subjects in a range usually considered pathological in healthy subjects. These results demonstrate that the responsiveness of the pituitary-adrenocortical system to the most important physiological stimuli, CRH and VP, is increased markedly in otherwise healthy subjects of old age.

According to the "glucocorticoid cascade hypothesis" adreno-cortical hypersecretion in the aged is partly caused by hippocampal damage. The hippocampus plays an important role in cognition and hippocampal damage is known to be associated with learning impairment and memory deficits. Patients with senile dementia of Alzheimer's type (SDAT) have serious hippocampal degeneration. From this one would expect that the disturbance of the BPA axis in SDAT patients is at least as pronounced as in mentally healthy subjects of comparable age. Therefore we studied the pituitary-adrenocortical response to stimulation

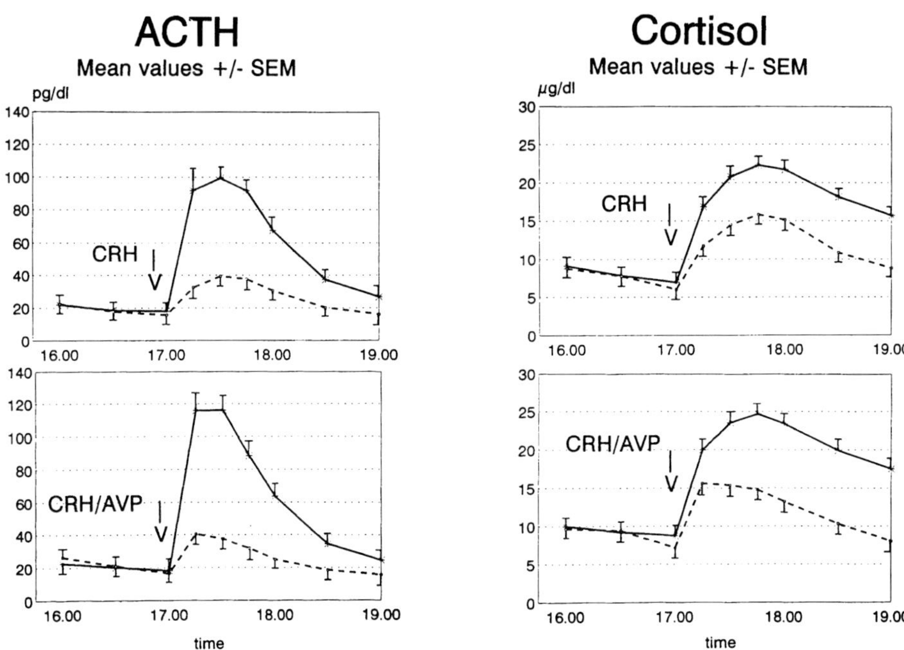

Fig. 2   Plasma ACTH and cortisol responses to stimulation with hCRH + AVP or hCRH alone in 10 healthy old subjects and in young controls. ACTH, adrenocorticotropic hormone; hCRH, human corticotropin releasing hormone; AVP, arginin-vasopressin.

with a combined bolus injection of hCRH and LVP in 3 groups of subjects [4]. Group A consisted of healthy male volunteers, age range 21−55 years, group B of mentally healthy elderly (mean age 74.5 years, age range 66−90 years, n = 15), group C of demented patients of the gerontopsychiatry unit who were otherwise healthy (mean age 75.2 years, age range 60−84 years, n = 12). Mean plasma cortisol and ACTH values before and after CRH/LVP administration are illustrated in Fig. 3. In case of cortisol, there were no significant differences during the baseline period. However, mentally healthy elderly exhibited higher mean peak cortisol levels than the young control group. Mean plasma ACTH levels during the baseline period were slightly, but significantly, increased in both groups of older patients. During the peak period, ACTH levels in the mentally healthy elderly were higher than those in young subjects or SDAT patients. This difference was maintained throughout the observation period of 120 minutes.

The striking result of this study is that the ACTH/cortisol responses to CRH/LVP in SDAT patients were not higher than those in young controls and, in contrast to expectation, lower than those in the age-matched controls. These findings argue against a major role of the hippocampus in causing the pituitary hyper-responsiveness characteristic of senescence. Why this hyper-responsiveness does not occur in SDAT patients remains to be elucidated.

In this study we also measured DHEA and DHEA-S levels. A distinct linear decrease in the plasma levels of these so-called adrenal androgens with age is well documented, leading to the postulate that DHEA or DHEAS is a discriminator of life expectancy and aging. More recently, Barrett-Connor et al. [1] demonstrated the DHEAS concentration is independently and inversely related to death from any cause and death from cardiovascular disease in men over 50 years. Finally, it has been claimed that plasma DHEAS concentrations are lower in patients with SDAT than in age-matched controls [22]. Our data are presented in Fig. 4. Mean DHEA levels of both groups of elderly were significantly lower than those in the young control group. However, there was no difference between demented and mentally healthy aged subjects. The same was true for DHEA-S levels [19].

The results discussed so far show that senescence is characterized by changes in the biosynthetic pathway of adrenal steroids within the adrenal gland, and by hyper-responsiveness of the pituitary-adrenal system to CRH and VP. This does not imply that there is enhanced BPA activity in physiological situations. Therefore, we examined the meal-related cortisol peak in a group of 11 old subjects (mean age 78 years, range 66−94 years). Again, old subjects showed significant elevated cortisol levels throughout the observation period when compared with a young controls. The magnitude of the cortisol increase was similar in both groups.

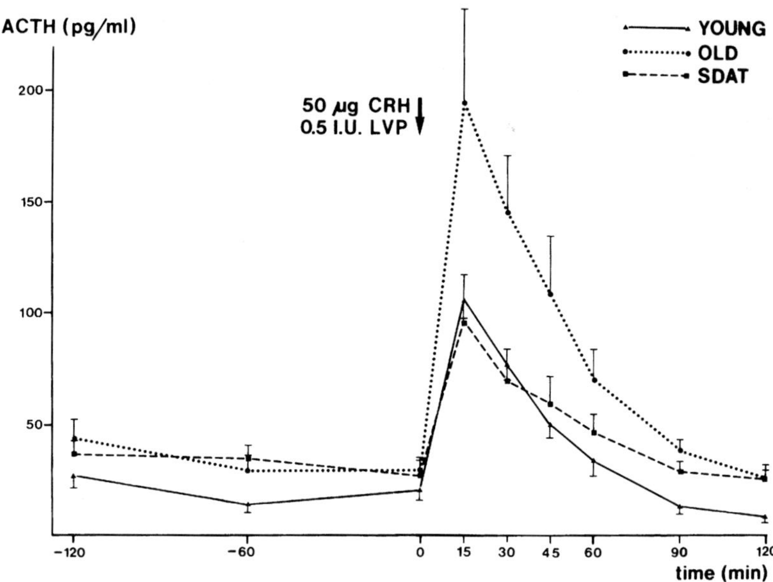

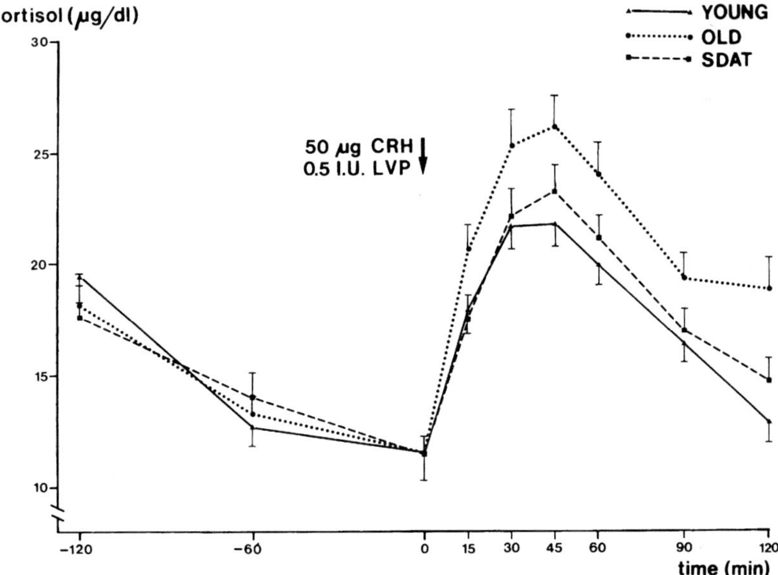

Fig. 3   Plasma ACTH and cortisol responses to hCRH + LVP in mentally healthy elderly, senile demented elderly (SDAT) and young persons to hCRH/LVP stimulation. ACTH, adrenocorticotropic hormone; hCRH, human corticotropin releasing hormone; LVP, lysin vasopressin.

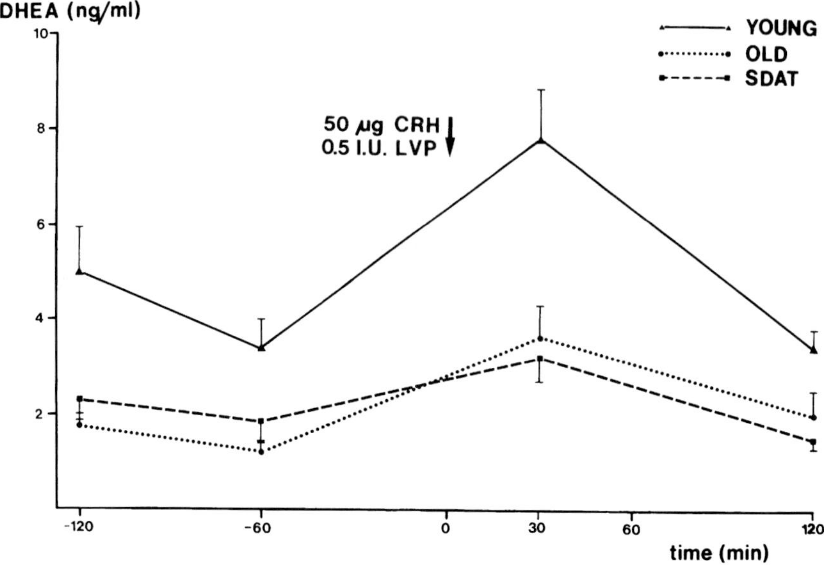

Fig. 4 Mean DHEA levels of young, mental healthy elderly, and senile demented elderly before and after stimulation with hCRH and LVP.

Nadir cortisol levels

Lesions of the hippocampus or fornix typically reduce diurnal variations in plasma corticosteroid levels, primarily by raising the nadir level toward that of the peak. This effect has been observed in a variety of species [10]. These data have frequently been interpreted to indicate that the hippocampus inhibits BPA activity primarily at the trough of the circadian rhythm.

In humans the nadir cortisol levels occur reliably during the first two cycles of nocturnal sleep [6]. By measuring plasma cortisol during sleep (sleep being monitored by polysomnography), it is possible to define exactly the individual cortisol nadir.

We used these methods to measure the plasma cortisol nadir in 28 subjects of different ages (20 years to 82 years). There was a significant positive correlation between the cortisol nadir and age ($r = 0.739$, $p < 0.001$) (Fig. 5). In an attempt to clarify whether this increase in the plasma cortisol nadir is due to a decreased number of hippocampal corticosteroid receptors, we blocked these receptors in young healthy subjects by pretreatment with the anti-mineralocorticoid canrenoate. In fact, after canrenoate, nadir and peak levels of plasma cortisol were increased as compared with the control session with placebo [5]. Thus, aging

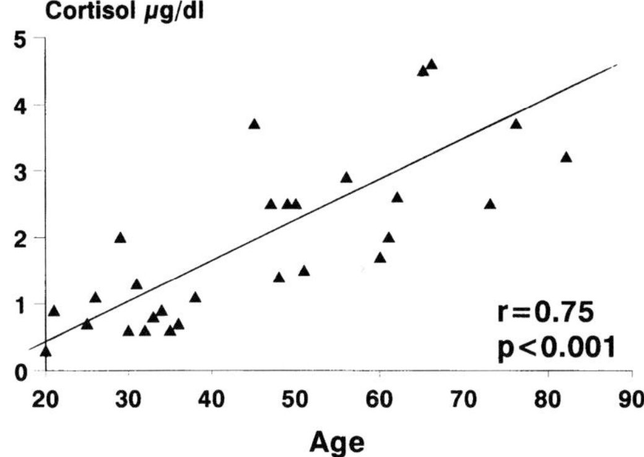

Fig. 5   Correlation of cortisol nadir levels with age in healthy subjects.

is accompanied not only by pituitary hyper-responsiveness, but also by increased nadir cortisol levels. The latter is presumably due to hippocampal damage.

CNS effect of ACTH and VP in the elderly

In extending the findings of D. de Wied's group in experimental animals, we demonstrated that in human beings also, peptides circulating in the peripheral blood can influence CNS functions [2]. In these experiments we found ACTH and ACTH fragments administered intravenously to impair selective attention. Selective attention was determined by comparing brain electrical responses evoked by tones when attented and when ignored, the difference between "attented" and "ignored" brain potential responses (Nd) representing a measure of selectivity of attention [9]. Vasopressin after intranasal application enhanced stimulus induced cortical arousal as measured by the so-called "vertex potential" [7].

Thus, the question arises whether age-related changes in the secretion of these peptide hormones contribute to the cognitive impairment characteristic for old age. In fact, selective attention is thought to be impaired with increasing age. There is one study in which selective attention was analysed utilizing the brain electrical responses to auditory stimuli in a dichotic listening paradigm [8]. Although the authors claim to have found no change in the Nd with age, scrutiny of their data shows diminished Nd's in the old subjects. Recent results from our laboratory demonstrate that the effect of intranasal VP on the vertex potential was diminished or even abolished in the elderly (Fig. 6).

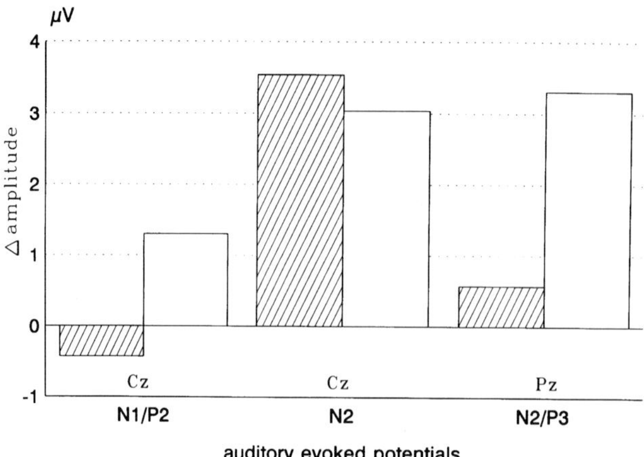

Fig. 6 Effects of intranasal administration of vasopressin on several components of auditory evoked potentials in young and old healthy subjects. The significant ($p < 0.05$) increase of the N1/P2 amplitude in young subjects was absent in the elderly. Similar results were obtained for the N2/P3 component. In case of the N2 component there was a significant vasopressin induced increase in both, old and young subjects.

These preliminary results demonstrate that not only the steroid hormones of the adrenal cortex, cortisol and DHEA, but also the peptide hormones of the BPA system, ACTH and VP, influence brain functions in the elderly and these influences can be profoundly different from those in young subjects.

Conclusions

Current concepts propose that aging is accompanied by and may result from disturbances in neuroendocrine functions, especially of the brain-pituitary-adrenocortical system. Our results obtained in human subjects of old age demonstrate age-related changes at the level of the adrenal gland, the pituitary, the hippocampus and of higher brain centers.

1. Biosynthetic pathways for glucocorticoid and adrenal androgens are differentially influenced by age.
2. At the pituitary level, hyper-responsiveness to various stimuli is demonstrable. The role of the hippocampus as cause of this phenomenon is unclear.
3. Basal cortisol secretion, especially the cortisol nadir, increases with age, presumably due to hippocampal disregulation.
4. Peptide hormones of the BPA system, ACTH and vasopressin influence higher brain functions in the elderly, and these influences can be profoundly different from those in young subjects.

References

[1] Barrett-Connor, E., Kay-Tee Khaw, S. C. C. Yen: A prospective study of dehydroepiandrosterone sulfate, mortality, and cardiovascular disease. N. Engl. J. Med. 315 (1986) 1519–1524.

[2] Born, J., H. L. Fehm: The hormonal modulation of stimulus processing in humans. Ger. J. Psychol. 12 (1987) 315–331.

[3] Cartlidge, N., M. Black, M. Hall et al.: Pituitary function in the elderly. Gerontol. Clin. 12 (1970) 65–69.

[4] Dodt, C., J. Dittmann, J. Hruby et al.: Different regulation of adrenocorticotropin and cortisol secretion in young, mentally healthy elderly and patients with senile dementia of Alzheimer's type. J. Clin. Endocrinol. Metab. 72 (1991) 272–276.

[5] Dodt, C., W. Kern, J. Born et al.: Antimineralocorticoid canrenoate enhances secretory activity of the hypothalamus-pituitary adrenocortical (HPA) axis in humans. J. Clin. Endocrinol. Metab., submitted.

[6] Fehm, H. L., J. Born: Evidence for entrainment of nocturnal cortisol secretion to sleep processes in human being. Neuroendocrinol. 53 (1991) 171–176.

[7] Fehm-Wolfsdorf, G., G. Bachholz, J. Born et al.: Vasopressin but not oxytocin enhances cortical arousal: an integrative hypothesis on behavioral effects of neurohypophyseal hormones. Psychopharmacol. 94 (1988) 496–500.

[8] Ford, J. M., R. F. Hink, W. F. Hopkins et al.: Age effects on event-related potential in a selective attention task. J. Gerontol. 34 (1979) 388–395.

[9] Hillyard, S. A., R. F. Hink, V. L. Schwent et al.: Electrical signs of selective attention in the human brain. Science 182 (1973) 177–180.

[10] Jacobsen, L., R. Sapolsky: The role of the hippocampus in feedback regulation of the hypothalamic-pituitary-adrenocortical axis. Endocrine Reviews 12 (1991) 118–134.

[11] Jensen, H. K., M. Blichert-Toft: Serum corticotropin, plasma cortisol and urinary excretion of 17-ketogenic steroids in the elderly (age group: 66–94 years). Acta Endocrinol. 66 (1971) 25–34.

[12] Meany, M. J., D. H. Aitken, C. van Berkel et al.: Effect of neonatal handling on age related impairments associated with hippocampus. Science 239 (1988) 766–768.

[13] Meites, J., R. Goya, Takahaski: Why the neuroendocrine system is important in aging processes. Exp. Gerontol. 22 (1987) 1–15.

[14] Pavlov, E. P., S. M. Harman, G. P. Chrousos et al.: Responses of plasma adrenocorticotropin, cortisol, and dehydroepiandrosterone to ovine corticotropin-releasing hormone in healthy aging men. J. Clin. Endocrinol. Metab. 62 (1986) 767–772.

[15] Sapolsky, R. M.: A mechanism for glucocorticoid toxicity in the hippocampus: increased neuronal vulnerability to metabolic insults. J. Neurosci. 5 (1985) 1228–1232.

[16] Sapolsky, R. M., L. C. Krey, B. S. McEwen: The neuroendocrinology of stress and aging: the glucocorticoid cascade hypothesis. Endocrine Reviews 7 (1986) 284–301.

[17] Sapolsky, R. M.: The adrenocortical axis. In: E. L. Schneider, J. W. Rowe (eds.): Handbook of the Biology of Aging, pp. 320–348. Academic Press, New York 1990.

[18] Sherman, B., C. Wysham, D. Pfohl: Age-related changes in the circadian rhythms of plasma cortisol in man. J. Clin. Endocrinol. Metab. 61 (1985) 439–443.

[19] Spath-Schwalbe, E., C. Dodt, J. Dittmann et al.: Dehydroepiandrosterone sulphate in Alzheimer disease. Lancet 335 (1990) 1412.

[20] Sunderland, T., C. R. Merril, M. G. Harrington: Reduced plasma dehydroepiandrosterone concentrations in Alzheimer's disease. Lancet ii (1989) 570.

[21] Waltman, C., M. R. Blackman, G. P. Chrousos et al.: Spontaneous and glucocorticoid-inhibited adrenocorticotropic hormone and cortisol secretion are similar in healthy young and old men. J. Clin. Endocrinol. Metab. 73 (1991) 495–502.

Function of the hypothalamo-pituitary testicular axis in elderly men

A. Vermeulen

Aging in males is accompanied by a decrease in total and even more so in free plasma testosterone concentration, and although the sequelae of chronic illness may accentuate this decrease, it is now generally accepted that even in healthy elderly males free testosterone levels are decreased [1].

There is strong evidence that this decrease has, to a larger extent, a primarily testicular origin. Indeed, it has been reported that the number of Leydig cells is decreased [2], that testicular perfusion is impaired [3], that the response of the Leydig cells to HCG stimulation is decreased in elderly males [4] and that the biosynthetic pathway is shifted towards the $\Delta4$ pathway [5]. Moreover, most authors observed increased levels of immunoreactive LH [4, 6−9], and although some authors reported that LH levels decreased [10], others observed increased LH levels in elderly men [11]. Finally, the LH response to classical GnRH stimulation appears to be unimpaired in elderly males [4, 10, 12].

Notwithstanding this rather convincing evidence for a primary peripheral origin, some observations do suggest that there also occur alterations at the hypothalamo-pituitary levels [11]. Indeed, the very fact that the decreased free testosterone levels are not compensated via increased LH stimulation suggests a resetting of the feedback sensor, and this is supported by the increased sensitivity to feedback by androgens in elderly men [13]. Moreover, the disappearance of the nycthemeral variations in plasma testosterone levels, most probably the consequence of alterations in LH release [14, 15], suggests alterations in the hypothalamo-pituitary compartment of the hypothalamo-pituitary gonadal axis.

We were interested in studying the effect of aging on the pulsatility of LH levels. We observed that under basal conditions, LH pulse frequency is similar in young and elderly males, but that the pulse amplitude is significantly decreased [16] in elderly men.

This decrease in amplitude could be the consequence of an increased estrogen level, of an increased opioid tone or of a decreased sensitivity of the gonadotrophs to GnRH. Estrogen levels however, are hardly increased in elderly men; moreover, if increased estrogen levels were responsible for the decreased LH pulse frequency, one would expect an increased effect of antiestrogens, which is not the case [17].

152   A. Vermeulen

As it is generally accepted that endogenous opioids have an inhibitory effect on the GnRH pulse generator, we considered the possibility that the decrease in LH pulse amplitude in elderly men was the consequence of an increased opioid tone. Therefore we administered a long acting oral antiopioid, Naltrexone, to both young and elderly men [16]. Whereas in young men naltrexone induced an increase, both in LH pulse frequency and pulse amplitude, no effect was seen on either parameter in elderly men [16]. Therefore it seems unlikely that the antiopioid tone in elderly men is increased, our data suggesting instead a decreased opioid tone.

Another possibility had to be considered, namely that the responsivity of the gonadotrophs to GnRH is decreased in elderly men. Although previous data have shown that the LH response to a maximal bolus dose of GnRH is not decreased in elderly men [4], the responsivity to small, physiological doses of GnRH, mimicking physiological stimulation, has not been studied.

Therefore we studied the responsiveness of the gonadotrophs by administering increasing doses of GnRH (from 0.625, 1.25, 2.5 and 5 µg administered as an I. V. bolus) with an interval of 120 minutes. The LH response to each dose, measured both as immunoreactive and biological activity, was similar in young and elderly men, excluding a decreased sensitivity of the gonadotrophs as a cause of the decreased LH pulse amplitude in elderly men.

The most likely explanation for the latter, therefore, is a decreased mass of GnRH released at each spontaneous pulse. Deconvolution analysis of spontaneous LH pulses showed that indeed the LH mass released at each pulse was significantly decreased in old age [18]. This is most easily explained by an age-associated reduction in cellular mass of the pulse generator.

The next question of course, is whether this decreased LH pulse amplitude has any consequence as far as Leydig cell function is concerned. Indeed, we know that pulsatile stimulation of the Leydig cells is not required in order to obtain an increase in testosterone secretion, as evidenced by hCG stimulation.

We observed, however, that there exists a significant linear correlation between mean plasma testosterone levels and both mean LH pulse amplitude and total pulse amplitude (Fig. 1), suggesting that the LH amplitude is indeed an important determinant of plasma testosterone levels.

In conclusion, if primary testicular alterations undoubtedly play a major role in the age-associated decline in Leydig cell function, it is now evident that alterations in hypothalamo-pituitary function, characterized by a decreased LH pulse amplitude, also play an important role.

Is there evidence that paracine factors play a role in the primary age-associated testicular alterations in Leydig cell function? It is generally acknowledged that

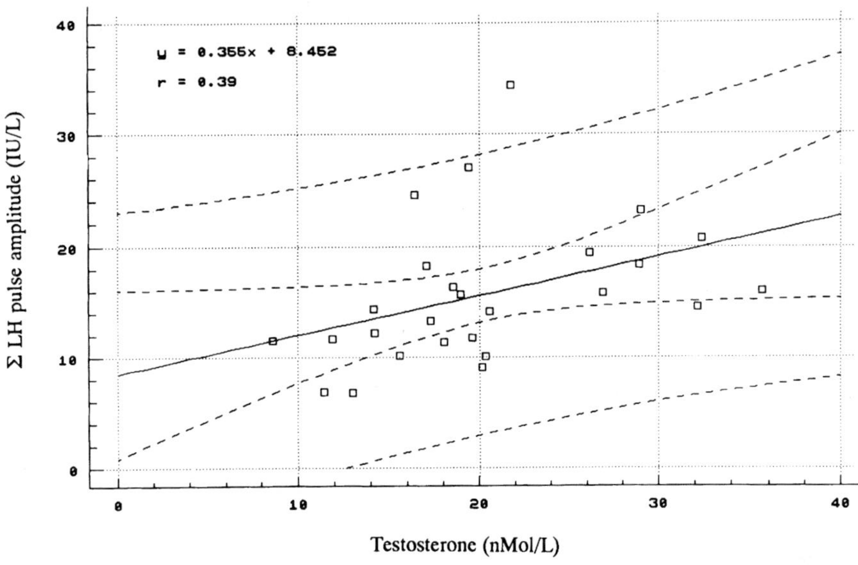

Fig. 1   Correlation between the sum of LH Pulse amplitudes and plasma testosterone levels in men 22−82 years old.

there exists a synergism between Leydig cell and Sertoli cell function, mediated by several paracrine factors, among which IgF-1 [19] and inhibin [20] are known to be capable, under certain conditions, of stimulating Leydig cell function. Evidently it is not possible to measure the local concentration of these paracrine factors which are active at the local, intratesticular level. Inhibin, however, is not only a paracrine factor but also a hormone, generally considered to be a marker of Sertili cell function, playing, together with the sex steroids, a major role in the regulation of FSH secretion.

Although no absolutely specific method for the determination of inhibin in plasma is available, an immuno-enzymatic method (Medgenix) allows the determination of inhibin in plasma with, however cross reaction with the α-subunit. Using this method, we observed that inhibin levels in normal males show a moderately pulsatile pattern (Fig. 2), and that there exists a highly significant correlation between variations in plasma LH and in plasma inhibin levels (P < 0.01) (Fig. 2). As LH pulses are generally considered to be largely correlated with FSH levels, this correlation is not unexpected. However, it is well known that LH, hCG and testosterone may also, by themselves, stimulate inhibin secretion, and that Leydig cells secrete an inhibin-like substance which, however, is biologically inactive.

In normal aging males, we observed an age-associated statistically highly significant decrease in plasma inhibin levels (Fig. 3), this notwithstanding the well

154   A. Vermeulen

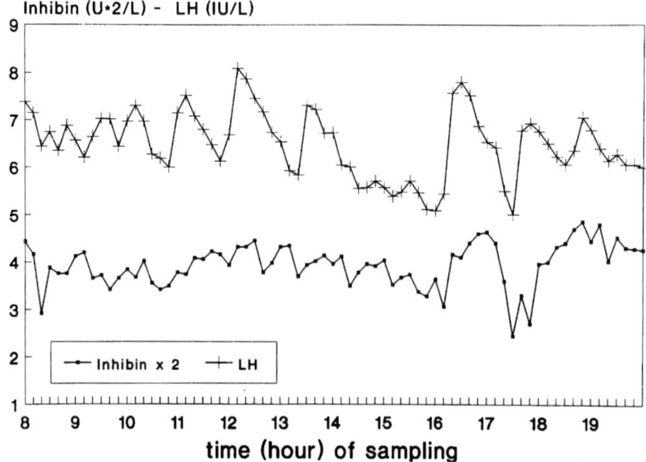

Fig. 2   Parallelism between plasma LH and inhibin levels in a normal man.

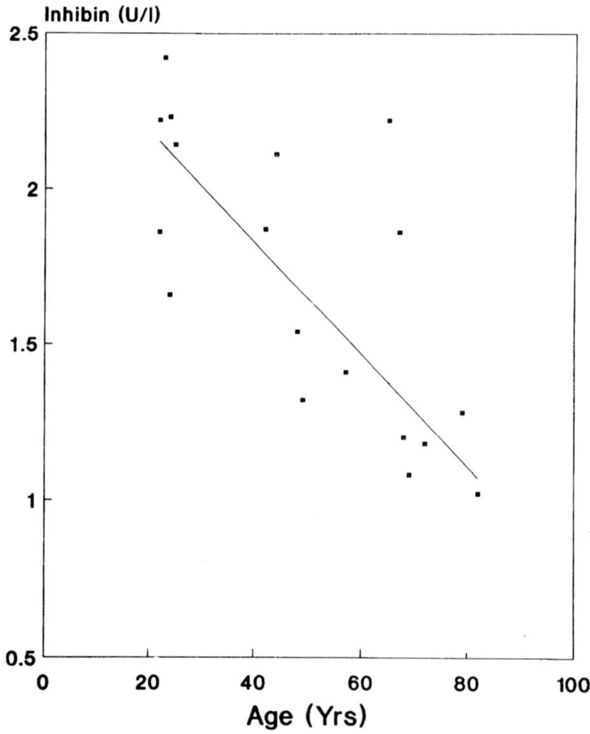

Fig. 3   Age dependent decrease of plasma inhibin levels in men.

known age associated increase in gonadotropin levels. A similar observation was made by Tenover et al. [21] and MacNaughton et al. [22].

Due to the interference of free α-subunits, these data should be interpreted cautiously, but these data certainly point towards an impaired Sertoli cell function in elderly males with decreased inhibin secretion, which might eventually play a role in the decreased Leydig cell function.

References

[1] Vermeulen, A.: Androgens and male senescence. In: E. Nieschlag, H. M. Behre (eds.): Testosterone, Action, Deficiency, Substitution, pp. 260−276. Springer Verlag, Berlin 1990.

[2] Neaves, W. B., L. Johnson, J. C. Porter et al.: Leydig cell numbers, daily spermproduction and serum gonadotrophin levels in aging men. J. Clin. Endocrinol. Metab. 59 (1984) 756−763.

[3] Suroanta, H.: Changes in small blood vessels of the adult human tests in relation to age: sample pathological conditions. Virchows Archiv (Path. Anat.) 51 (1971) 508−512.

[4] Rubens, R., M. Dhont, A. Vermeulen: Further studies on Leydig cell function in old age. J. Clin. Endocrinol. Metab. 39 (1974) 40−47.

[5] Vermeulen, A., J. P. Deslypere: Intratesticular unconjugated steroids in elderly men. J. Steroid Biochem. 24 (1986) 1079−1083.

[6] Isurugi, K., K. Fukutani, H. Takayasu et al.: Age related changes in serum luteinizing hormone (LH) and follicle stimulating hormone (FSH) levels in normal men. J. Clin. Endocrinol. Metab. 39 (1974) 955−957.

[7] Baier, H. G., K. J. Buro: Serum levels of FSH, LH and testosterone in human males. Horm. Metab. Res. 6 (1974) 514−516.

[8] Harman, S. M., P. D. Tsitouras, P. F. Costa et al.: Reproductive hormones in aging men. II. Basal pituitary gonadotropins and gonadotropin responses to luteinizing hormone releasing hormone. J. Clin. Endocrinol. Metab. 51 (1982) 547−551.

[9] Lungmayr, G., J. Spona: Hypophysäre und gonadale Funktionsreserve des Mannes in Abhängigkeit vom Alter. Wiener Klin. Wschr. 87 (1975) 200−204.

[10] Urban, R. J., J. D. Veldhuis, R. N. Blizzard et al.: Attenuated release of biologically active luteinizing hormone in healthy aging men. J. Clin. Invest. 81 (1988) 1020−1029.

[11] Tenover, J. S., A. M. Matsumoto, S. R. Plymate et al.: The effects of aging in normal men on bioavailable testosterone and luteinizing hormone secretion: response to clomiphene citrate. J. Clin. Endocrinol. Metab. 65 (1987) 1118−1126.

[12] Baker, H. W. G., H. G. Burger, D. M. de Kretser et al.: Endocrinology of aging: pituitary testicular axis. Proc. of the 5th congr. of Endocrinol. 2 (1977) 479−485.

[13] Winters, S., R. J. Sherins, P. Troen: Gonadotropin suppressive activity of androgens is increased in elderly men. Metabolism 33 (1984) 1052−1059.

[14] Bremner, W. J., M. V. Vitello, P. N. Prinz: Loss of circadian rhytmicity in blood testosterone levels with aging in normal men. J. Clin. Endocrinol. Metab. 56 (1983) 1278−1281.

[15] Deslypere, J. P., A. Vermeulen: Leydig cell function in normal men: Effect of age life style, residence and activity. J. Clin. Endocrinol. Metab. 59 (1984) 955−962.

[16] Vermeulen, A., J. P. Deslypere, J. M. Kaufman: Influence of antiopioids on luteinizing hormone pulsatility in aging men. J. Clin. Endocrinol. Metab. 68 (1989) 68−72.

[17] Tenover, J. S., W. J. Bremner: The effects of normal aging on the response of the pituitary gonadal axis to chronic clomiphene administration in men. J. of Androl. 12 (1991) 253−257.

[18] Kaufman, J. M., M. Giri, J. P. Deslypere et al.: Influence of age on the responsiveness of the gonadotrophs to luteinizing hormone − releasing hormone in males. J. Clin. Endocrinol. Metab. **72** (1991) 1255−1260.

[19] Verhoeven, G., J. Cailleau: Influence of coculture with Sertoli cells on steroidogenesis in immature rat Leydig cells. Molecul. Cellul. Endocrinol. **71** (1990) 239−251.

[20] Hsueh, A. J. W., K. D. Dahl, J. Vanghan et al.: Heterodimers and homodiners of inhibin subunit have different paracrine action in the modulation of luteinizing hormone stimulated androgen biosynthesis. Proc. Nat. Acad. Sc. **84** (1987) 5082−5086.

[21] Tenover, J. S., R. J. McLachlan, K. D. Dahl et al.: Decreased serum inhibin levels in normal elderly men: evidence for a decline in Sertoli cell function with aging. J. Clin. Endocrinol. Metab. **67** (1988) 455−459.

[22] MacNaughton, J., M. L. Bangah, P. I. McCloud et al.: Inhibin and age in men. Clin. Endocrinol. **35** (1991) 341−346.

Diabetes mellitus in the elderly

W. Kerner

Prevalence of diabetes in the elderly

About 3.5 million people in Germany, almost 4 percent of the population, report having diagnosed diabetes [16]. Although this estimate is for diabetes of all types, 90 to 95 percent of people older than 30 with diabetes probably have non-insulin dependent diabetes (NIDDM). This figure underestimates the true number of patients with this disease because a considerable proportion of all adult diabetes cases are undiagnosed and therefore not reported. When both diagnosed and undiagnosed diabetes cases are counted, the true prevalence of the disease is even greater. In the United States, half of diabetes cases [11], and in Germany approximately one–third [4], are undiagnosed. This means that true diabetes prevalence in Germany will be 4.5 to 5 million cases or 5.5 to 6 percent of the population. Diabetes prevalence increases with increasing age. Prevalence in the Framingham Study is 3 to 5 percent in people between 50 and 59 years of age, about 10 percent in people between 60 and 69 years and 10 to 15 percent in people older than 70 years [30]. In the United States, prevalence of diagnosed diabetes in individuals over 65 years of age increased from 4 to 10 percent during the last decade [15]. This increase is due in part to an increasingly aged population and to decreasing mortality from cardiovascular disease.

Macrovascular disease in elderly diabetic patients

Coronary heart disease (CHD), peripheral vascular disease and cerebrovascular disease are more common, occur at an earlier age and tend to be more extensive in diabetic patients of both sexes. Several studies show a 2 to 4-fold increase in CHD mortality in male NIDDM patients compared with the general population [9]. Some studies have reported a greater increase in coronary heart disease mortality among women with NIDDM. As with CHD, the risk of stroke is increased 2 to 5-fold among NIDDM patients [3, 25]. The excess risk, if any, for females is less pronounced than in the case of CHD. Data from the Framingham Study show a 4 to 6-fold increased incidence of intermittent claudication in diabetic men and women [12]. When peripheral vascular disease is diagnosed by Doppler flow measurement its prevalence has been found to be 7-fold higher in NIDDM patients than in control subjects [2]. Diabetes is an independent risk factor for atherosclerotic cardiovascular disease, increasing risk 2 to 3-fold [28]. Other major risk factors — hypertension, high cholesterol levels and cigarette smoking — increase mortality caused by cardiovascular disease in people with diabetes to a similar extent as in people without diabetes. Hypertension is frequently observed in patients with NIDDM. The prevalence of hypertension is 1.5 to 2-fold higher in NIDDM patients than in control subjects [30]. Lipid abnormalities occur frequently in NIDDM patients. The characteristic pattern of dyslipidemia consists of hypertriglyceridemia and low HDL-cholesterol. Reported prevalences of hyperlipidemia vary greatly from 15 to 50 percent [9], depending on the characteristics of the study population, including level of obesity, glycaemic control, medications, and thyroid and renal diseases.

There is overwhelming evidence for a high prevalence of cardiovascular disease at the time of diagnosis in NIDDM patients [10]. The same observation is made for the prevalence of hypertension and hyperlipidemia at the time of diagnosis. Therefore, atherosclerotic diseases in NIDDM patients may not represent "late complications" as in the case of microvascular complications. It has been suggested that NIDDM is from the beginning a syndrome characterized by glucose intolerance, obesity, hyperlipidemia and hypertension (Syndrome X, Metabolic Syndrome, Deadly Quartet) [13]. This view is supported by the observation that mortality from cardiovascular diseases does not strictly correlate with duration of NIDDM [29].

Prognosis of diabetes in elderly patients

Diabetes is associated with an increased mortality at all ages [8, 20]. Overall mortality rates are approximately twice as high as in non-diabetic subjects. Excess mortality declines consistently with increasing age at diabetes onset. Death rates of patients who were > 75 years old at time of diagnosis are not significantly different from non-diabetic individuals [21]. Interestingly, overall mortality rates in female NIDDM patients exceed or equal those in males. Cardiovascular diseases comprise the major causes of death in patients of both sexes with NIDDM. They account for 60 to 70 percent of the deaths in these patients. A small proportion of deaths in this group (< 5 percent) are caused by renal disease, with the remainder due to all other causes [7].

Neurologic complications and amputations

Pain from neuropathy is a common complaint among diabetic patients. A recent study found that over a one-year period, 76.8 percent of diabetic subjects aged

60 to 70 years complained of lower extremity pain, as compared with 38.7 percent of control subjects [6]. Published studies on the epidemiology of lower extremity amputations in diabetic individuals do not differentiate between different types of diabetes [18, 27]. However, in patients older than 65 years, most of them presumably suffering from NIDDM, risk of amputation is 5 to 17-fold higher than in control subjects. Amputation in patients with diabetes is associated with peripheral vascular disease and/or neuropathic complications and may be precipitated by minor trauma. Risk factors for amputation are impaired circulation, absence of lower leg vibratory perception, low HDL-cholesterol levels, and a lack of previous diabetes education [24].

Microvascular complications

Contrary to common belief, retinopathy is frequent in older patients with diabetes. The Framingham Study found that 19 percent of patients aged 55 to 84 years had retinopathy [23]. In patients older than 75 years prevalence was more than 25 percent. Senile macula degeneration, open-angle glaucoma and senile cataracts also increse in incidence with age, and are increased in diabetic patients [17]. Diabetes (IDDM and NIDDM) is responsible for 8 percent of legal blindness in the United States [7]. It is estimated that 5.5 percent of those with diabetes diagnosed at 60 years of age become blind after 20 years of diabetes [7]. The prevalence of retinopathy in old patients increases with the duration of diabetes [14].

Diabetes is the most common cause of end-stage renal disease. The risk of end-stage renal disease is about 10-fold lower for patients with NIDDM than for those with IDDM (0.5 percent during 10 years of observation in NIDDM, 5.8 percent in IDDM) [5]. However, due to the much higher prevalence of NIDDM, in most dialysis centers a considerable number of elderly patients with diabetes are treated. It is well documented that development and progression of nephropathy is associated with hypertension.

In summary, diabetes in the elderly is associated with an increased overall mortality as a consequence of the higher prevalence of cardiovascular diseases. Symptoms of CHD, peripheral vascular disease and non-fatal stroke impair the quality of life in a considerable proportion of these patients. In addition, more elderly patients with diabetes suffer from blindness, end-stage renal disease, amputation and painful neuropathy than non-diabetic subjects of the same age group.

Diagnosis of diabetes in the elderly

The symptoms characteristic of IDDM (polyuria, polydipsia, weight loss) are rarely present in elderly patients with newly manifested diabetes. NIDDM typically causes no symptoms for many years and the onset and progression of symptoms can be slow. Sometimes, complaints from neuropathy or retinopathy, cardiovascular disease or urinary tract infection are the first symptoms of long-standing disease.

According to the criteria of the National Diabetes Data Group, diabetes is diagnosed [19] in nonpregnant adults who have one of the following:

1) random plasma glucose level of 200 mg/dl or greater and classic signs and symptoms of diabetes mellitus; or
2) fasting plasma glucose of 140 mg/dl on at least two occasions; or
3) fasting plasma glucose less than 140 mg/dl plus sustained elevated plasma glucose levels during at least two oral glucose tolerance tests. The 2-hour sample and at least one other between zero and two hours after 75 g glucose dose should be 200 mg/dl or greater.

The WHO criteria for diagnosis of diabetes [31] are similar: Diabetes is likely in persons with random venous plasma glucose over 200 mg/dl. Diagnosis of diabetes is established by a fasting plasma glucose over 140 mg/dl or a plasma glucose over 200 mg/dl two hours after a 75 g oral glucose load.

Both criteria are not age-related but conservative enough to exclude age-related deterioration of glucose tolerance. It has been shown that fasting plasma glucose levels increase by one mg/dl per decade after the age of 50 years in the non-diabetic elderly population. The 2-hour plasma glucose level in a glucose tolerance test rises by approximately 10 mg/dl per decade. Therefore, age-related deterioration of glucose tolerance will result in most individuals in the diagnosis not of diabetes but of impaired glucose tolerance. This condition is defined in WHO criteria by a fasting plasma glucose below 140 mg/dl and a plasma glucose between 140 and 200 mg/dl two hours after a 75 g oral glucose load. Impaired glucose tolerance may be associated with an increased risk of cardiovascular disease, but it does not predispose to diabetic microvascular or neuropathic complications.

As soon as diabetes has been diagnosed, diseases typically associated with diabetes must be searched for: hypertension, coronary heart disease, peripheral vascular disease, neuropathy, diabetic foot lesions, retinopathy, nephropathy.

Therapy of diabetes in the elderly

It is important to recognize that treatment strategies in elderly patients with diabetes must be individualized on 1) the basis of functional ability, 2) the presence of associated and coexisting diseases and 3) life expectancy. In addition, treatment should improve, not impair, the quality of life in these patients.

The basic principles of therapy discussed below have to be modified for each patient according to his or her individual needs.

Hyperglycemia is generally treated in the same way as in younger patients with NIDDM, starting with a trial of diet first, followed by use of oral hypoglycemic agents and ultimately insulin when diet and tablets fail.

The diet for elderly patients with diabetes is not substantially different from those for younger patients. In obese patients, weight reduction should be achieved by moderate restriction of caloric intake (usually 1000 to 1200 kcal/ day). Dietary instructions should be simple and individualized to the patients' habits. It is important to define for each individual a realistic goal for weight reduction to be achieved within a period of several months. Weight loss regularly results in reduction of hyperglycemia, lowering of elevated blood pressure and improvement of hyperlipidemia. However, weight reduction is difficult at any age and success rates are especially low for old people.

Exercise should be used as an adjunct to other forms of therapy for diabetes in the elderly. However, these people frequently face limitations to exercise, including cardiovascular disease, limited joint mobility, proliferative retinopathy, neuropathy and peripheral vascular disease.

Treatment with sulfonylurea drugs is commonly started when dietary therapy is unsuccessful. The indication for this therapy should be regularly reevaluated over time. The most serious risk of the use of sulfonylurea drugs is the development of hypglycemia, sometimes with fatal outcome. Besides increasing age, the risk of developing hypoglycemia is increased by a previous history of stroke or cardiovascular disease, an impaired renal function, decreased food intake, diarrhea, alcohol ingestion and interaction with other drugs, particularly sulfonamides [1]. Patients with significant renal failure should not be treated with sulfonylurea drugs.

The presence of diseases which represent contraindications for the use of metformin usually prohibits the use of this drug in elderly people with diabetes.

Insulin therapy should be started when therapy with oral hypoglycemic agents fails. Most olderly patients respond satisfactorily to a mixture of NPH and regular insulin injected once or twice daily. The major side effect of insulin is hypoglycemia, which is particularly undesirable in old people with impaired cerebral function. In elderly patients who have poor dexterity and visual or cognitive impairment, drawing up and injecting insulin preparations may be difficult. This problem can be ameliorated by the use of special injection devices (insulin pens).

In elderly diabetic patients, diabetes education is as important as in younger patients. Education must be adapted to the individual capabilities and needs of the patients. Education programs will mainly deal with dietary instructions, insulin injection technique, prevention and treatment of hypoglycemia and prevention of diabetic foot lesions. Most patients will benefit from urine glucose monitoring, some from blood glucose monitoring.

There are no generally valid blood glucose goals in elderly patients with diabetes. These goals mainly depend on the patients' physical condition and his or her life expectancy. In addition, the increased risk associated with hypoglycemia in elderly patients with cardiovascular and cerebrovascular disease must be weighed against the desire to achieve near-normoglycemia. It is generally accepted that long-standing hyperglycemia is the main cause of diabetic microvascular and neuropathic complications. Therefore, near-normoglycemia must be the therapeutic goal in elderly patients with relatively high life expectancy because these patients are at risk of develping such complications during their lifetime. The life expectancy of a woman 70 to 74 years old is 13.9 years. Taking into account that patients with NIDDM may have had the disease many years before diagnosis, a 72-year old woman with newly diagnosed diabetes is at risk of developing diabetic complications [12]. On the other hand, in an 85-year-old patient with newly diagnosed diabetes, it may be sufficient to lower blood glucose until symptoms of hyperglycemia are corrected. It is sometimes argued that elderly patients with diabetes will not benefit from near-normoglycemia because their life expectancy is not reduced when diabetes is diagnosed at old age. Although there is in fact no convincing evidence that lowering glucose reduces morbidity and mortality from cardiovascular diseases, this argument does not take into consideration the fact that development of microvascular and neuropathic complications will markedly impair the quality of life in these patients.

Hypertension is frequently associated with diabetes in the elderly and contributes to increased mortality from cardiovascular diseases. General measures for treatment of hypertension include weight reduction, avoidance of alcohol, restriction of sodium intake, and physical activity. Selection of appropriate drugs for treatment of hypertension in elderly people with diabetes is mainly determined by the presence of coexisting diseases (CHD, cardiac failure, obstructive lung disease, peripheral vascular disease, renal failure). First-line agents are beta-blockers, diuretics, ACE-inhibitors, calcium-antagonists and postsynaptic alpha-blockers. Therefore, in contrast to the hypertension in IDDM patients, an ACE-inhibitor must not always be the drug of first choice in older diabetic patients. Therapy of hypertension should aim at a blood pressure below 140/90 mmHg in younger patients with NIDDM, and below 160/90 mmHg in older patients. Recent data obtained in non-diabetic subjects suggest that treatment of isolated systolic hypertension in old patients (above 60 years) reduces the risk of stroke [26].

Hyperlipidemia, another risk factor for atherosclerosis, is frequently present in old patients with diabetes. As for non-diabetic elderly individuals, it is not generally accepted that reduction of cholesterol levels influences morbidity and mortality from cardiovascular diseases. Angiographic studies have demonstrated that lipid-lowering can induce regression of atherosclerotic lesions in coronary arteries. Large controlled trials will be necessary to demonstrate a possible effect of lipid-lowering on mortality in elderly patients with established atherosclerotic disease.

References

[1] Asplund, K., B. E. Wilholm, F. Lithner: Glibenclamide-associated hypoglycemia: a report on 57 cases. Diabetologia 24 (1983) 412–417.

[2] Beach, K. W., G. R. Bedford, R. O. Bergelin et al.: Progression of lower-extremity arterial occlusive disease in type II diabetes mellitus. Diabetes Care 11 (1988) 464–472.

[3] Biller, J., B. B. Love: Diabetes and stroke. Med. Clin. N. Am. 77 (1993) 95–110.

[4] Bormann, C., J. Hoeltz, H. Hoffmeister et al.: Subjektive Morbidität. Beiträge des Bundesgesundheitsamtes zur Gesundheitsberichterstattung II. MMV MedizinVerlag München 1990.

[5] Cowie, C. C., F. K. Port, R. A. Wolfe et al.: Disparities in incidence of diabetic end-stage renal disease according to race and type of diabetes. N. Engl. J. Med. 321 (1989) 1074–1079.

[6] Damsgaard, E. M.: Why do elderly diabetics burden the health care system more than nondiabetics. Dan. Med. Bull. 36 (1989) 89–92.

[7] Diabetes 1993. Vital Statistics. American Diabetes Association 1993.

[8] Goodkin, G.: Mortality Factors in Diabetes. J. Occup. Med. 17 /1975) 716–721.

[9] Haffner, S. M., M. P. Stern, M. Rewers: Diabetes and Atherosclerosis: Epidemiological considerations. In: B. Draznin, R. H. Eckel (eds.): Diabetes and Atherosclerosis: Molecular basis and clinical aspects, pp. 229–254. Elsevier, New York 1993.

[10] Hanefeld, M., S. Fischer, H. Schmechel et al.: Diabetes intervention study: Multi-intervention trial in newly diagnosed NIDDM. Diabetes Care 14 (1991) 308–317.

[11] Harris, M. I.: Undiagnosed NIDDM: Clinical and Public Health Issues. Diabetes Care 16 (1993) 642–652.

[12] Kannel, W. B., D. L. McGee: Diabetes and cardiovascular disease. The Framingham Study. J. Am. Med. Assoc. 241 (1979) 2035–2038.

[13] Kaplan, N. M.: The deadly quartet. Upper-body obesity, glucose intolerance, hypertriglyceridemia, and hypertension. Arch. Int. Med. 149 (1989) 1514–1520.

[14] Klein, R. R.: The epidemiology of diabetic retinopathy. In: J. Pickup, G. Williams (eds.): Textbook of diabetes, pp. 557–563. Blackwell Scientific Publications, Oxford 1991.

[15] Krolewski, A. S., J. H. Warram: Epidemiology of Diabetes Mellitus. In: Joslin's Diabetes mellitus, 12th edition, pp. 12–42. Lea & Febiger, Philadelphia 1985.

[16] Michaelis, D.: Zur Praevention des Diabetes mellitus unter Berücksichtigung epidemiologischer und ätiopathogenetischer Aspekte. Z. Ges. Inn. Med. 40 (1985) 473–479.

[17] Morse, P. H.: Ocular symptoms and signs of diabetes. Geriatrics (1976) 59–63.

[18] Most, R. S., P. Sinnock: The epidemiology of lower extremity amputations in diabetic individuals. Diabetes Care 6 (1983) 87–91.

[19] National Diabetes Data Group: Classification and diagnosis of diabetes mellitus and other categories of glucose intolerance. Diabetes 28 (1979) 1039–1057.

[20] Panzram, G., R. Zabel-Langhennig: Prognosis of diabetes mellitus in a geographically defined population. Diabetologia 20 (1981) 587−591.
[21] Panzram, G.: Mortality and survival in Type 2 (non-insulin-dependent) diabetes mellitus. Diabetologia 30 (1987) 123−131.
[22] Peters, A., M. B. Davidson: Aging and Diabetes. In: K. G. M. M. Alberti, R. A. DeFronzo, H. Keen, P. Zimmet (eds.): International Textbook of Diabetes mellitus. Volume 2, pp. 1103−1149. John Wiley & Sons, Chichester−New York−Brisbane−Toronto−Singapore 1992.
[23] Podgor, M. J., M. C. Leske, F. Ederer: Incidence estimates for lens changes, macular changes, open-angle glaucoma and diabetic retinopathy. Am. J. Epidemiol. 118 (1983) 206−212.
[24] Reiber, G. E., R. E. Pecoraro, T. D. Koepsell: Risk factors for amputation in patients with diabetes mellitus. A Case-Control Study. Ann. Int. Med. 117 (1992) 97−105.
[25] Roehmholdt, M. E., P. J. Palumbo, J. P. Whisnant et al.: Transient ischemic attack and stroke in a community-based diabetic cohort. Mayo Clin. Proc. 58 (1983) 56−58.
[26] SHEP Cooperative Research Group: Prevention of stroke by antihypertensive drug treatment in older persons with isolated systolic hypertension. Final results of the systolic hypertension in the elderly program (SHEP). J. Am. Med. Assoc. 265 (1991) 3255−3264.
[27] Siitonen, O. I., L. K. Niskanen, M. Laakso et al.: Lower-extremity amputations in diabetic and non-diabetic patients. A population-based study in eastern Finland. Diabetes Care 16 (1993) 16−20.
[28] Stamler, J., O. Vaccaro, J. D. Neaton et al.: Diabetes, other risk factors, and 12-Yr cardiovascular mortality for men screened in multiple risk factor intervention trial. Diabetes Care 16 (1993) 434−444.
[29] Vigorita, V. J., G. W. Moore, G. M. Hutchins: Absence of correlation between coronary arterial atherosclerosis and severity or duration of diabetes mellitus of adult onset. Am. J. Cardiol. 46 (1980) 535−542.
[30] Wilson, P. W. F., K. M. Anderson, W. B. Kannel: Epidemiology of diabetes mellitus in the elderly. The Framingham Study. Am. J. Med. 80 (1986) 3−9.
[31] World Health Organization: WHO Expert Committee on Diabetes Mellitus. Second Report. WHO, Geneva, 1980.

Osteoporosis

R. Ziegler

Bone mass: dependency on sex hormones and aging

The human bone mass depends on unalterable factors such as inheritance and aging as well as alterable factors: nutrition, hormones, and physical activity (Fig. 1). Although inheritance cannot be influenced for an individual, it can be of medical importance for the next generation: a daughter of an osteoporotic patient will be more intensively advised at the age of menopause to take estrogen replacement therapy (ERT) than a women without such history.

The three alterable factors are of essential importance for the optimal development and maintenance of bone mass — if one of them is defective, the genetically determined peak bone mass will not be reached, or there will be an earlier or faster loss. In part, the factors can compensate for each other: e.g. physical activity may overcome the consequence of mild undernutrition. On the other hand, a certain hierarchy of the factors is evident: the excess of physical exercise (sports) which leads to secondary hypogonadism does not balance the bone loss due to insufficient sex hormones. In other words: among the essential factors, sex hormones are still more important than too much exercise.

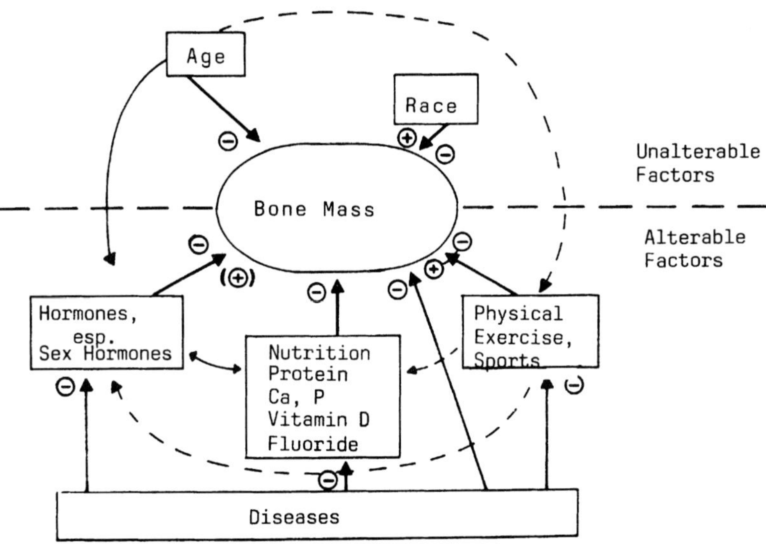

Fig. 1   Factors which influence bone mass.

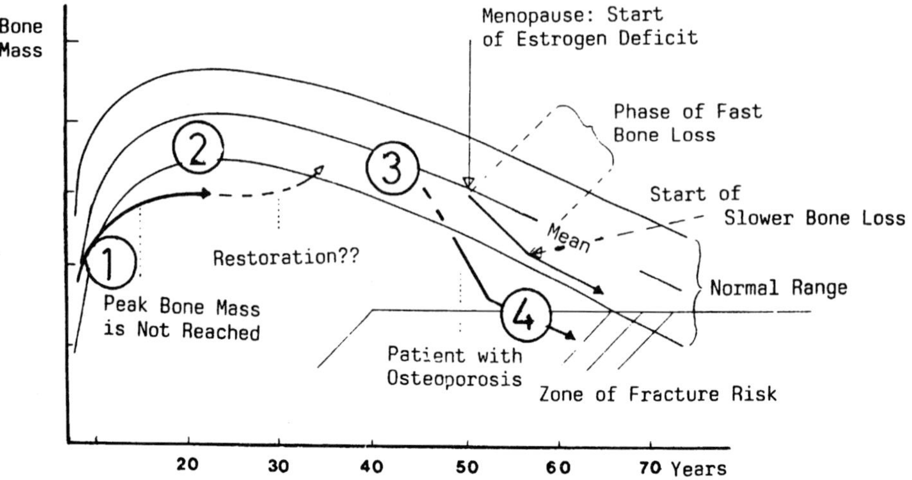

Fig. 2   The course of bone mass during life, depending on the presence of sex hormones. The numbers indicate points of intervention (see text).

Fig. 2 depicts course of bone mass during life, especially under the aspect of sex hormone supply. Children's bones grow without needing sex hormones; however, at the time of puberty they suddenly become sex hormone dependent — the reasons for this sensitivity are unknown. If puberty does not happen in time, peak bone mass will not be built up. Female ballet dancers who had a delayed menarche suffered from much more bone fractures than those having there menarche in time [34]. The hope for catch-up bone growth to reach peak bone mass somewhat later, after some years of adequate hormone supply, is perhaps not justified, as shown in hypogonadal men: if testosterone substitution started later than 17−20 years of age, peak bone mass was never reached [5].

If secondary hypogonadism starts later in life, bone loss happens as after menopause. Patients suffering from anorexia or hyperprolactinemia over years present with lower bone mass [1, 27]. As mentioned above, excess sports do not produce better bone mass as soon as they lead to amenorrhea as a signal of hypoestrogenism [8].

Fig. 2 shows that peak bone mass declines after the 30th or at least 40th year of life. Even in the healthy individual there is an annual bone loss of ½ to one percent of bone mass per year. This loss may be delayed by exercise [22]. In the male, the bone loss curve of aging will parallel the curves of the function of other organs such as heart, lungs, and even testicles: the senile man has of course lower testosterone levels than the younger man at the time of his peak bone mass. There are no data published on what would happen to male bone mass in cases of persistently high testosterone levels — the risk of an increase in prostate cancer would speak against such studies.

In the female, menopause happens around the age of 50. The fall in endogenous estrogens is followed by a period of 6—8 years of accelerated bone loss; the biochemical events are discussed below. In case of low peak bone mass, early menopause, and fast loss over too many years, osteoporosis will develop presenting with vertebral (trabecular cone) fractures at the age of 60 to 70. This condition is named postmenopausal or type I osteoporosis [24]. Fractures of the more compact bones such as the distant radius and/or femoral neck in general happen later in life (70 to 80 years of age) — they characterize senile or type II osteoporosis [24]. It is noteworthy that fractures at senility are less determined by low bone mass than by the additional risk of falling due to impaired eyesight, hearing capacity, reaction speed or even soft tissue thickness above the hip [4].

Prophylaxis of osteoporosis by sex hormones

For the physician, the prevention of the development of osteoporosis starts in a patient's childhood and continues throughout. General recommendations refer to optimal lifelong calcium supply throughout his or her life [32]. The same is true for exercise.

The endocrinologist has the special task watching, over the optimization of sex hormones. The first point of intervention (see Fig. 2) is at the time of puberty: If puberty does not take place spontaneously at the right time, hormone substitution should be considered. A delayed start may prevent the development of optimal peak bone mass. Young girls exercising for ballet or sports who obviously postpone their menarche, should reduce their training program. If this reasonable option is rejected because of the patient's (or parent's) eagerness, at least ERT should be initiated as a primary prevention of osteopenia or osteoporosis.

The second point of intervention (Fig. 2) is longer lasting secondary amenorrhea. Respective conditions are: anorexia mentalis, status after ovarectomy (if there is no contraindication against ERT), pituitary insufficiency. Again, in case, of excessive sports leading to amenorrhea, the training program should be reduced. If this is not done, ERT is indicated.

The third intervention point (Fig. 2) is relevant for all women because they pass the natural fate of menopause. Physicians and gynecologists should consider

ERT if there is a risk for later osteoporosis evident. The decision requires a detailed family and personal history, an exact physical examination and, bone mineral densitometry (BMD) and/or x-rays mostly of the spine. BMD alone is not adequate as there is a broad overlap between healthy people and osteoporotics. Risk factor lists are worked out [33].

The fourth point of intervention is not prevention, but treatment of manifest osteoporosis after fracturing and after a period without estrogens (see next paragraph).

Treatment of overt osteoporosis based on pathophysiology

How estrogens protect the bone against resorption and thus maintain bone mass is not yet fully explained. After deprivation of estrogens, a chain of changes takes place in calcium homeostasis and bone metabolism which ends in the loss of bone mass (Fig. 3). In the absence of estrogens, osteolysis is increased at lower concentrations of resorptive agents such as parathyroid hormone (PTH). This sensitization of the bone cells has not yet been analyzed. Suggestions that a lack of endogenous calcitonin may explain the increased resorption were not definitely confirmed.

The increase in osteolysis leads to a mild increase of serum calcium within the normal range − there is no hypercalcemia. Nevertheless, PTH levels fall and thus less calcium is reabsorbed in the kidney: increased serum calcium and diminished reabsorption result in an additional calcium daily excretion of about 30 mg calcium [11]. Per year this means the loss of 1% of the skeletal calcium via urine which doubles the normal loss in the presence of the sex hormones. In some women the loss may be even greater ("fast loser"): up to 10% of trabecular bone may be lost during the first postmenopausal year [6].

PTH is also an important stimulator of the formation of calcitriol (1,25-dihydroxycholecalciferol) out of calcidiol in the kidneys. Due to lower PTH levels in blood, hypoestrogenic women will produce less calcitriol − the consequence is diminished calcium absorption from the gut. This will be deleterious, especially in cases of poor calcium supply e. g. when low calorie diets are adopted to maintain a too-slim body shape. The combination of increased resorption with increased urinary calcium loss and diminished calcium utilisation ends in decreased bone mass as a prerequisite for osteoporotic fractures. Unexplained is the individual risk: all women pass menopause, but only a minority (exact percentages are not yet known for Germany; current epidemiological studies will hopefully yield the figures) will develop osteoporosis with fractures. Is the initial peak bone mass more decisive than the later loss? Is fast loss the responsi-

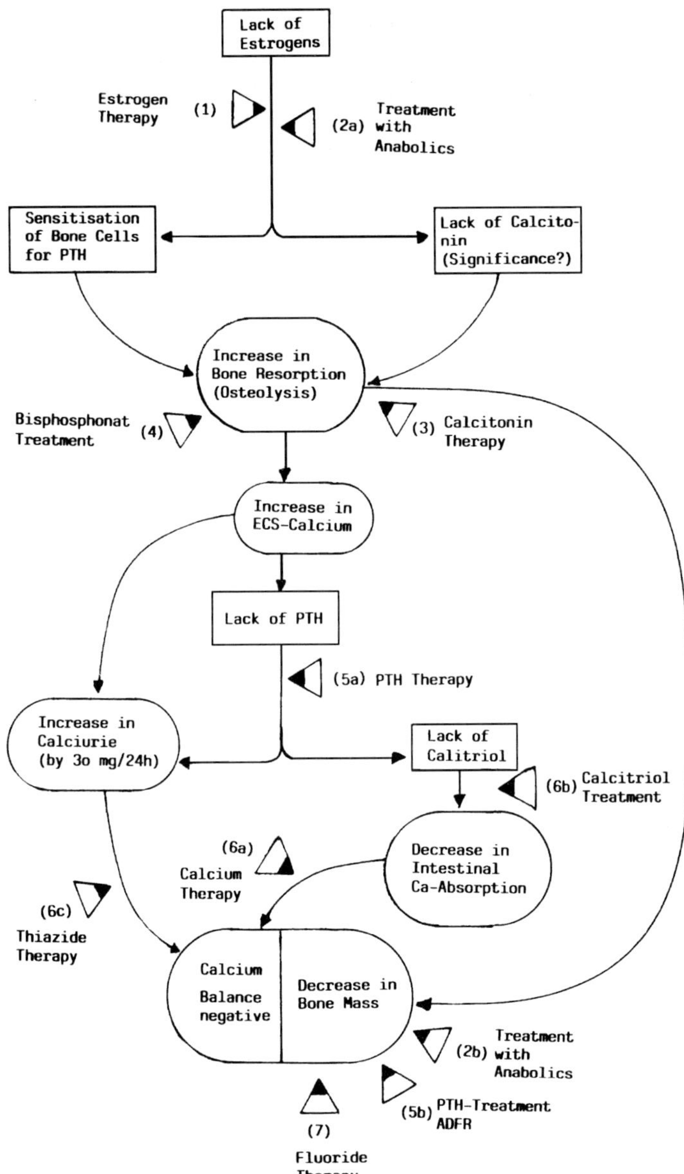

Fig. 3 Pathophysiology of osteoporosis: the numbered arrows indicate the points of intervention (see text).

ble defect which is perhaps genetically determined? It was interesting to learn that children from female as well as male osteoporotics have lower bone mass in younger years [28].

The numbers in Fig. 3 indicate where interventions are tried or considered at the moment. The term "antiresorptive treatment" is used for all agents which reduce the activity of osteoclasts (Point 1). Estrogens are the most physiological substitutive antiresorptive treatment. They are (like all antiresorptives) more efficient as higher bone turnover goes on. During the later and slower phase of bone loss ("low turnover"), about 10 to 15 years after menopause, estrogen-dependent bone loss plays only a minor role, and the percentage of conserved bone will be lower than in the fast loss condition.

Anabolics as modified androgens act like sex hormones, i. e. on one hand as a substitutive agent (Point 2a). On the other hand, they may exert additional effects on the muscles ("body-builder"-effect) supporting new bone formation (Point 2b).

Calcitonin inhibits the activity of the osteoclasts, therefore it acts as an antire-sportive agent (Point 3). Whether this treatment is substitutive or pharmacody-namic is an unanswered theoretical question.

Bisphosphonates (Point 4) are chemicals which block bone resorption. Primarily they were considered within ADFR-schemes according to the suggestions by Frost [10]: Activation of bone turnover should be achieved by e. g. PTH (or thyroid hormones), depression of resorption by calcitonin or bisphosphonates should prevent exaggerated bone loss, formation of new bone should take place by the osteoblasts which were activated via coupling, repetition of the cycle should begin when osteoblast activity calms down after some weeks to months. It turned out that the bisphosphonate etidronate was equally efficient whether there was a preceding activation (phosphate administration in order to stimu-late endogenous PTH) or not [35].

PTH (Point 5a) was considered as a substitutive agent [14], on the other hand it was considered as an osteoanabolic stimulator according to the ADFR-con-cept (Point 5b).

Calcium therapy (Point 6a) is substitutive like calcitriol (Point 6b) − it may be partially antiresorptive: whereas premenopausal women need about 1000 mg calcium per day in order to maintain neutral calcium balance, women without estrogens require 1500 mg calcium for this purpose [13]. Their bone loss is then delayed, although not as much as in the case of ERT. Nevertheless, calcium supply = treatment is often underestimated. The administration of thiazide diuretics (Point 6c) which diminish calciuria is an alternative to oral calcium supply e. g. in patients with recurrent renal stone disease [17].

Osteogenetic or osteoanabolic treatment tends to increase bone mass beyond the possibilities to stop (increased) resorption. The low turnover situation of the bone tissue especially favors the use of agents which directly stimulate the osteoblasts. Besides the already mentioned principles like PTH and ADFR

(Point 5b) and the anabolic steroids (Point 2b), fluorides proved to be very efficient activators of the osteoblasts (Point 7). Presumably fluoride ions prolong the activity of local growth factors [9]. Futural aspects refer to the use of such growth factors especially considering the fact that a latent lack of growth hormone and factor activity may contribute to the development of osteoporosis. However such speculations are still far from practical application.

Efficiency of medical treatment

Effective treatment of osteoporosis is not documented merely by an increase in bone mass, but also proof of stability, i. e. the end of further fracturing is required. Up to now, an abundance of publications reported on bone mass measurements whereas data regarding fractures are limited.

Antiresorptives: estrogens

Many retrospective studies show that women on ERT have fewer osteoporotic fractures than women without substitution [12]. However, mostly pure estrogens were used in the past, and data on the currently used estrogen/progestagen-combination are limited. However, as progestagens also influence bone in a positive manner and, as first randomized studies also show, produces a lower fracture incidence under such conditions [18] (Fig. 4), ERT can be regarded as an effective treatment. But the exact number of spared fractures is not yet known.

Anabolic steroids

There are only limited data that anabolics slightly increase and then maintain bone mass [7]. A study with small numbers of patients [15] also shows lower fracture rates (Fig. 4).

Calcitonin

Calcitonin is very efficient in preventing postmenopausal bone loss [20]. In case of osteoporosis its effectiveness depends on initial bone metabolism: in cases of high turnover an increase in bone mass takes place, whereas bone mass does not change in cases of low turnover [3]. In a recent study [2] a decrease in fractures is also reported − however, the control collective on calcium shows a very low fracture incidence which limits the generalization of such findings (Fig. 4).

Bisphosphonates

Several bisphosphonates proved to prevent bone loss. However, fracture data were only published for etidronate. The Danish study [30] showed no statistical

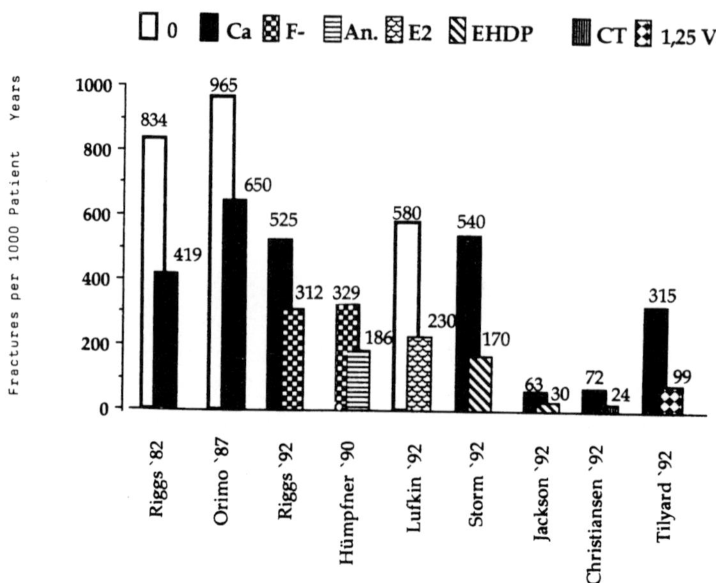

Fig. 4 Fracture rates and influence of different therapeutic agents. Notice the big differences of the studies in the calcium arms! Abbreviations: O = no treatment; Ca = calcium; F^- = fluorides; An = anabolics; E_2 = estrogens; EHDP = etidronate; CT = calcitonin; 1,25 VitD = calcitriol.

difference between calcium- and calcium-plus etidronate-treated women over three years, but the difference was significant if the second and third years were analyzed. The overall fracture rate of 5 years (170 fractures per 1000 patient's years) was lower than that of the calcium treated rate over three years (540/ 1000 years) [29]. The parallel USA-study (15) showed a 50% lower fracture rate during two years compared to calcium treatment (30 vs. 63 fractures per 1000 years); after an increase of fractures during the third year (116) the fourth year showed again the low frequency of 30 fractures per 1000 years [16]. There was no difference in the increase in bone mass whether phosphate activation was performed before etidronate or not. Further studies are, of course, desired, especially because the fracture numbers in the calcium arms of the studies differ enormously [Fig. 4].

Calcium

Retrospective studies already showed some years ago that calcium treatment reduced vertebral fracture rates to about half of untreated controls [26] (Fig. 4). However, such studies were not randomized like later ones [21] which had the disadvantage of small numbers. Later studies do not compare calcium treatment with no treatment because it is considered to be unethical not to treat with at least calcium. Therefore the question for us of current studies is whether there is an agent more efficient than calcium (which has to be optimized with respect to its dosage). Recently it was shown that calcitriol may be more efficient than calcium alone to diminish fracture rates [31]. However, in this study the question whether vitamin D alone would exert the same activity as calcitriol remained unanswered.

Osteoanabolic treatment: ADFR

As already mentioned, etidronate treatment was performed with and without preceding activation of bone turnover, but there were no differences. When PTH activation was combined with calcitonin depression, the scheme induced an increase in bone mass by 26% during 14 months [14]. Fracture rates were not reported, and some of the treated had no diminished bone mass.

Fluorides

As mentioned, do fluorides stimulate bone formation. In contrast to other agents, F^- continues the increase in bone mass during the third and fourth year of treatment [31]. The data on fracture rates are conflicting: The study of the Mayo Clinics [23] showed a 15% lower fracture rate in women treated with NaF plus calcium compared with calcium treatment alone, but the difference was not statistically significant. In contrast, the French study [19] showed statistically significant fewer fractures during fluoride treatment. Recently, the Mayo data were followed and analyzed further [25]. If the disadvantages of the study design (uncoated tablets with fast fluoride release, no intended lowering of dosage in case of side effects) were drawn into consideration, optimal fluoride doses in fact reduced vertebral fracture rate (Fig. 4). As with the other drugs, further data are required for fluoride, especially in comparison with other agents.

Conclusions

Osteoporosis is a disease which is in many cases, especially in the female, related to natural hypogonadism at menopause. Prevention has to be considered lifelong from puberty to menopause. After fractures estrogens have to be considered as adiuvants to other principles of treatment. The lack of estrogens leads to other endocrine phenomena such as (perhaps) low calcitonin, low PTH, and low calcitriol. All these hormones are tried for substitutive, antiresorptive treatment. Potent chemical antiresorptives are the bisphosphonates. To overcome diminished bone formation at low turnover, osteoanabolic treatment is desired. ADFR-schemes including PTH are challenging, but still empiric efforts.

Anabolic steroids may exert effects beyond sex hormone substitution by increasing muscle mass and strength. As chemical agents fluorides stimulate osteoblasts — presumably they increase the activity of local growth factors. Altogether, the presently used drugs for the treatment of overt, fracturing osteoporosis do not yet fulfil the requirements of differentiated treatment — the respective data are not comparable to each other. Therefore, a randomized study comparing several agents, such as the project "Osteoporose 2000", [36] are mandatory.

References

[1] Cann, C. E., M. C. Martin, H. K. Genant et al.: Decreased spinal mineral content in amenorrheic women. JAMA **251** (1984) 626−629.

[2] Christiansen, C., K. Overgaard: Clinical use of salmon calcitonin — new findings. Workshop on osteoporosis. Florence, Italy, April 23−24, 1992.

[3] Civitelli, R., S. Connelli, F. Zacchei et al.: Bone turnover in postmenopausal osteoporosis. Effect of calcitonin treatment. J. Clin. Invest. **82** (1988) 1268−1274.

[4] Cooper, C., C. Wickham, K. Walsh: Appendicular skeletal status and hip fracture in the elderly: 14-year prospective data. Bone **12** (1991) 361−364.

[5] Cordes, U., G. Kurz, S. Kapp: Der verspätete Einsatz einer Hormonsubstitutionstherapie verhindert bei hypogonaden Männern das Erreichen einer maximal möglichen Knochenmasse. In: G. Willert, F. H. W. Heuck (Hrsg.): Neuere Ergebnisse in der Osteologie, pp. 95−106. Springer-Verlag, Heidelberg 1989.

[6] Dambacher, M. A., J. Ittner, P. Rüegsegger: Osteoporose — Pathogenese, Prophylaxe, Therapie. Internist **27** (1986) 206−213.

[7] Dequeker, J., P. Geusens: Anabolic steroids and osteoporosis. Acta Endocrinol. [Suppl.] **271** (1985) 45−52.

[8] Drinkwater, B. L., Nilson, K., C. H. Chesnut III et al.: Bone mineral content of amenorrheic and eumenorrheic athletes. New Engl. J. Med. **311** (1984) 277−281.

[9] Farley, J. R., N. M. Tarbaux, S. L. Hall et al.: Evidence that fluoride-stimulated ^{3}[H]-thymidine incorporation in embryonic chick calvarial cell cultures is dependent on the presence of a bone cell mitogen, sensitive to changes in the phosphate concentration, and modulated by systemic skeletal effectors. Metabolism **37** (1988) 988−995.

[10] Frost, M. M.: Osteopenia: the ADFR treatment. In: B. Frame, J. J. Potts jr. (eds.): Clinical disorders of bone and mineral metabolism. Excerpta Medica, Amsterdam−Oxford−Princeton. ICS **617** (1983) 368−374.

[11] Gallagher, J. C., B. E. C. Nordin: Oestrogens and calcium metabolism. In: van Keep, P. A., C. Lauritzen (eds.): Oestrogens and aging, Karger, Basel 1973.

[12] Gordan, G. S., J. Picchi, B. S. Roof: Anti-fracture efficacy of long-term estrogens for osteoporosis. Trans. Ass. Amer. Phys. **86** (1973) 326−332.

[13] Heaney, R. P.: Optimizing bone mass in the perimenopause: Calcium. In: M. Kleerekoper, S. M. Krane (eds.): Clinical disorders of bone and mineral metabolism, pp. 181−187. Mary Ann Liebert Inc. Publ., New York−Basel 1989.

[14] Hesch, R. D., E. F. Rittinghaus, H. M. Harms et al.: Die Frühtherapie der Osteoporose mit (1-38) Parathormon und Calcitonin-Nasalspray. Med. Klinik **84** (1989) 488−498.

[15] Hümpfner, A., W. Schulz: Therapie der primären Osteoporose mit dem Anabolikum Stanozol: eine Alternative zu Natriumfluorid? Proceedings of the 6th annual meeting of the section

calciumregulating hormones and bone metabolism of the German Society of Endocrinology, pp. 51−62. Heidelberg 5th October 1990.

[16] Jackson, R. D., S. T. Harris, H. K. Genant et al.: Cyclical etidronate treatment of postmenopausal osteoporosis: 4 year experience. Bone Min. **17** (Suppl. 1), Abstrakt 316 (1992) 154.

[17] LaCroix, A. Z., J. Wienpahl, L. R. White et al.: Thiazide diuretic agents and the incidence of hip fracture. New Engl. J. Med. **322** (1990) 286−290.

[18] Lufkin, E. G., H. W. Wahner, W. M. O'Fallon et al.: Treatment of postmenopausal osteoporosis with transdermal estrogen. Ann. Int. Med. **117** (1992) 1−9.

[19] Mamelle, N., P. J. Meunier, R. Dusan et al.: Risk-benefit ratio of sodium fluoride treatment in primary vertebral osteoporosis. Lancet **13** (1988) 361−365.

[20] Mazzuoli, G. F., S. Tabolli, F. Bigi et al.: Effects of salmon calcitonin on loss of bone mass induced by ovariectomy: controlled double blind study. In: G. F. Mazzuoli (ed.): Calcitonin '88, pp. 15−24. Sandoz AG, Basel 1989.

[21] Orimo, H., M. Shiraki, T. Hayashi et al.: Reduced occurrence of vertebral crush fractures in senile osteoporosis treated with $1\alpha(OH)$-vitamin D_3. Bone Min. **3** (1987) 47−52.

[22] Prince, R. L., M. Smith, I. M. Dick et al.: Prevention of postmenopausal osteoporosis. A comparative study of exercise, calcium supplementation, and hormone-replacement therapy. New Engl. J. Med. **325** (1991) 1189−1195.

[23] Riggs, B. L., S. F. Hodgson, W. M. O'Fallon et al.: Effect of fluoride treatment on the fracture rate in postmenopausal women with osteoporosis. New Engl. J. Med. **322** (1990) 802−809.

[24] Riggs, B. L., L. J. Melton: Involutional osteoporosis. New Engl. J. Med. **314** (1986) 1676−1686.

[25] Riggs, B. L., W. M. O'Fallon, S. F. Hodgson et al.: Clinical trial of fluoride in osteoporotic women: extended observation and additional analyses. Bone Min. **17** (Suppl. 1), Abstract 20 (1992) 74.

[26] Riggs, B. L., E. Seemann, S. F. Hodgson et al.: Effect of the fluoride/calcium regimen on vertebral fracture occurrence in postmenopausal women. New Engl. J. Med. **306** (1982) 446−450.

[27] Rigotti, N. A., R. M. Neer, S. J. Skates et al.: The clinical course of osteoporosis in anorexia nervosa. JAMA **265** (1991) 1133−1138.

[28] Seeman, E., J. L. Hopper, L. A. Bach et al.: Reduced bone mass in daughters of women with osteoporosis. New Engl. J. Med. **320** (1989) 334−338.

[29] Storm, T., G. Thamsborg, G. Kollerup et al.: Five years of intermittent, cyclical etidronate therapy increases bone mass and reduces vertebral fracture rate in postmenopausal osteoporosis. Bone Min. **17** (Suppl. 1), Abstrakt 328 (1992) 157.

[30] Storm, T., G. Thamsborg, T. Steiniche et al.: Effect of intermittent cyclical etidronate therapy on bone mass and fracture rate in women with postmenopausal osteoporosis. New Engl. J. Med. **322** (1990) 1265−1271.

[31] Tilyard, M. W., G. F. S. Spears, J. Thomson et al.: Treatment of postmenopausal osteoporosis with calcitriol or calcium. New Engl. J. Med. **326** (1992) 357−362.

[32] Toss, G.: Effect of calcium intake vs. other life-style factors on bone mass. J. Int. Med. **231** (1992) 181−186.

[33] van Hemert, A. M., J. P. Vandenbroucke, J. C. Birkenhäger et al.: Prediction of osteoporotic fractures in the general population by a fracture risk score: J. Epidemiol. **132** (1990) 123−135.

[34] Warren, M: P., J. Brooks-Gunn, L. H. Hamilton et al.: Scoliosis and fractures in young ballet dancers. Relation to delayed menarche and secondary amenorrhea. Engl. J. Med. **314** (1986) 1348−1353.

[35] Watts, N. B., S. T. Harris, H. K. Genant et al.: Intermittent cyclical etidronate treatment of postmenopausal osteoporosis. New Engl. J. Med. **323** (1990) 73−79.

[36] Ziegler, R.: Das Dilemma der Osteoporose-Therapie. Dt. Ärzteblatt **87** (1990) A847−A849.